CREATIVE HEALING

CREATIVE
HEALING

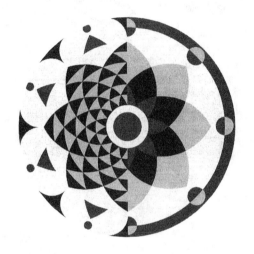

HOW TO HEAL
YOURSELF BY TAPPING YOUR
HIDDEN CREATIVITY

MICHAEL SAMUELS, M.D.
and **MARY ROCKWOOD LANE, R.N., Ph. D.**

RESOURCE *Publications* · Eugene, Oregon

Resource Publications
A division of Wipf and Stock Publishers
199 W 8th Ave, Suite 3
Eugene, OR 97401

Creative Healing
How to Heal Yourself by Tapping Your Hidden Creativity
By Samuels, Michael, MD and Lane, Mary Rockwood, RN, PhD
Copyright©1998 by Samuels, Michael, MD
ISBN 13: 978-1-61097-045-7
Publication date 10/14/2010
Previously published by HarperSanFrancisco, 1998

From Mary:
To my sweet family, David, Anneliese, Francesco, and Tim.

◆　　◆　　◆

From Michael:
To my family, Lewis and Rudy, and Nancy, who is with us in spirit.

CONTENTS

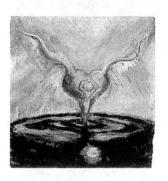

ACKNOWLEDGMENTS

We would like to thank all of the wonderful artists who have shared their healing work with us. Their spirits are alive in this book in their words and in their images. We would like to thank Elaine Markson, our agent, for continuing to be a beacon of light guiding our work. We thank Mark Chimsky, our editor, for a heroic, thoughtful, and careful edit. We thank Katie Carlin for her hard work in helping us edit this large book; Sally Hutchinson, Carol Reed Ash, and Sandy Seymore for their support with Mary's Ph.D. on art and healing; Marshall and Phyllis Klaus for talking about our book and sharing theirs. Mary would like to thank Albert Alcalay for being the most wonderful influence and mentor, Jerry Cutler for his support of her painting, and her dear friend Lee Ann Stacpoole for being the artist who encouraged her to heal herself with art. Mary would also like to thank Meredith Wellman for her wonderful dedication in taking care of her children while she worked on this book. Michael would like to thank James Surls for taking him up on the mountain to have the vision of art and healing as one. Michael would like to thank Marion Weber for funding Art As A Healing Force for three years. We would like to thank Linda Samuels for her work on the Art As A Healing Force slide library and her help in illustrating this book, and Mimi Farina for her magnificent *Bread and Roses.* Mary would like to thank Melanie Sorensen for her lifelong friendship. We both would like to thank Dr. John Graham-Pole for his untiring leadership in the field of arts and medicine and Christiane Corbat for being the healing artist extraordinaire.

Branham Rendlen, *Open Hearted.* The heart open and flying is one of our symbols of art and healing. Branham says, "Art has definitely been a healing force in my life. The work has been instrumental in my own healing from trauma I experienced as a child. As I have communicated with my innermost self through image, imagination, and symbol, I have experienced a form of soul retrieval. Through the artwork, I have come to understand myself as a part of this energy that heals, is creativity and love."

My paintings entered me into a very deep healing process. They were powerful, a powerful door to help me conquer a virus that had taken over my body. I was directed to paint each color, each image, each pattern, from a different voice within, a part of me that was fighting for my life. Every painting in the series took me on a unique journey that informed me of another part to the healing process. The painting and I became one, until it was time to move on. I was moved by my art through an illness that forever changed my life.

—Denise Bardovi, about healing herself
of chronic fatigue syndrome by painting

◆　◆　◆

My friend who was a nurse called me to please come down to the hospital. So I brought T-shirts with me and some paints and things. She said, "We have a little girl here who has been waiting to see you. I told her you were coming." She was seven years old. I had never been on a bone marrow transplant unit. I looked through the window and she was so excited. This little girl was all tied up to her intravenous lines. She was jumping up and down—straight up and down—that I was there, and clapping her hands when I walked in. The nurse told me that she had been standing at the window and looking out waiting for me to come all day. And she was just like, "Are you gonna play with me, are you gonna do this with me, are you gonna—can we paint?"

—Mary Lisa Kitakis, an artist-in-residence,
about her first day in the hospital

◆　◆　◆

The creative healing process is like a pot becoming fired. It is like making a pot with soft clay that is your previous life. It is soft, pliable, capable of infinite molding. In the fire it becomes formed and stable and you become strong. And then you make more pots to share with the world in love. You are changed forever.

—Mary Rockwood Lane, about the
lived experience of being an artist healer

Art as a Passionate Way of Healing

Oh daylight rise! Atoms are dancing
Souls, lost in ecstasy, are dancing.
I'll whisper in your ear where the
dance will take you.
All atoms in the air, in the desert,
They are all like madmen, each atom,
happy or miserable,
Is Passionate for the sun
of which nothing can be said.

Rumi

Creative Healing is a book about freeing your inner healer by embracing the passionate creative artist that is within each of us. It is a book about healing yourself, others, or the earth by tapping into the creative energy that makes us and keeps us alive.

PRAYER, ART, AND HEALING

Prayer, art, and healing all come from the same source: the human soul. Research has shown us that a person in prayer, a person making art, and a person healing all have the same physiology, the same brain wave patterns, and the same states of consciousness. *Creative Healing* is about conquering illness and healing body and soul. In this book, when we use the word *art*, we speak of all the creative arts. This includes the visual arts, painting, sculpture, photography, and crafts. You can heal yourself with writing, poetry, journals, essays, stories, storytelling, or theater. Music, songs, tones, chanting, silence, sounds of nature, and dance, movement, ritual, circle dancing, and ecstatic dance all are deeply healing. Art in *Creative Healing* is all creativity; it is any way we can be creative in our lives.

Art and healing is a new medically proven technique that strengthens body, mind, and spirit. Art and healing can help you to heal illnesses, including cancer, AIDS, and depression. It can help you reduce symptoms, alleviate pain, and improve your attitude and the quality of your life. *Creative Healing* is not only about healing; it is also a spiritual path. It can help you feel connected to others and the earth. We want *Creative Healing* to be accessible to everyone. We believe that everyone is an artist, and everyone can be an artist healer if they want to be. It is a way of being, a way of seeing, a way of drawing, a way of making music, a way of writing, and a way of dancing that is deeply personal and transformative. When we say prayer, art, and healing all come from the same source, we mean that they are three paths coming together as one. The parts of each of us that are spiritual, that are creative, and that are self-healing or healers all come together in this sacred process. They join, explode, and change us and the world.

Creative Healing is not only about one healing modality; it is about freeing the healer within. It is not about being a certain kind of artist; it is about you being the most creative person that you can be. It is not about one spiritual path; it is about luminosity. It is about honoring yourself and waking up the creative spirit inside of you and letting that spirit come forth. It is about being an artist as a healer, for that is who you are. We have tried to make *Creative Healing* a deeply personal book. Think of it as a conversation. Much of it is taken from conversations between the authors about art and healing and from interviews with people in this field. It is very real; it is not abstract. We are reminding you that what you know about art and healing is already deep inside of you. It is within all of us; it is our inheritance and birthright.

This book is an invitation to you. It provides the support, tools, and suggestions for how to heal yourself or others with art. *Creative Healing* takes something you do every day and turns it into a spiritual path for going even deeper into the spiritual center of your life. Follow us inward to your heart. Let art, writing, music, and dance heal you and transform your life.

AN INVOCATION FOR OUR HEALING WORK TO BE BLESSED

Healers in many traditions pause for a moment and center themselves or say a prayer before they heal or make art. We would like to honor this practice and call on our helping forces before starting our work together.

> *As we start this journey, let us pray to those who are with us to help us on the way. Let us pray for them to come to us and be with us in this work we are about to do. God, Buddha, Great Spirit, Our Teachers, She Who Gardens Us from Above, come to us and help us with this work. We thank you for the earth, for our families, and for us as the artists that we all are. We thank you for our spirits and our ability to pray, to make art, and to heal. We thank you for our eyes, our ears, our hands, our bodies, and our lives. Help us tell the truth and help us understand these words. Help us heal ourselves, others we love, and the earth. Help us make art and healing one.*

If you wish, close your eyes a moment and be silent. Pause and center yourself. Thank the powers that you believe in; pray for what you need. Now we will start our work together.

NANCY'S STORY

Nancy was a forty-six-year-old woman with breast cancer. One day after carpooling and making lists of errands for the church and school committees, while she was preparing dinner and rushing around the house, she received a phone call from her doctor telling her that her routine mammogram needed repeating. When she went to the breast clinic, she was worried, but she was still focused on her life of working, carpooling, and going to meetings. In the doctor's office she was quickly told that the needle biopsy of her breast lump looked malignant and that she would get the results the next day. She left the office dazed and frightened. Suddenly she saw her whole life as if it were behind a huge shimmering dark veil that blocked the sun and kept her from seeing her world. She spent the next days deep in fear, depression, and darkness. The biopsy showed breast cancer, and she was told that she needed to have surgery, radiation, and chemotherapy.

As time went on, Nancy realized that she needed to recreate her life. As she came to understand the seriousness of her situation, she also realized that her life was now different and that she had to do things to make it hers. The endless errands and responsibilities seemed increasingly empty to her as she looked around for ways to heal herself of her breast cancer. She went to therapists, changed her diet, and started to exercise. But she knew that all these treatments were from "outside of her" and could not by themselves change her life. Listening to her intuition, she went deep inside herself and looked to what she loved the most. She started by visiting with her friends and talking to them about her life and theirs. She found she wanted long, slow lunches without time pressure in a space that was just hers. From this choice she knew what was next. She remembered in what place she was most at peace … it was in her garden. She remembered the long hours spent pruning her apple trees at dusk, with her babies playing under the trees. So she reclaimed the one thing that was meaningful to her—the astonishing beauty of gardens. She went from the space of illness to elsewhere, to the passionate space inside of her that was in love with the flowers. She went to her soul's center, where she saw her husband and her children perfectly, in total compassion and love.

Next she visited nearby gardens and read gardening books. Her bedside was piled high with books filled with lush colors and long vistas. As she took chemotherapy, she talked with her physician about which English gardens were most exciting to visit. She visited garden experts and ate lunch with them and planned trips to special English gardens that had flowers in borders she wanted to see. She went to nurseries and studied plants that she was attracted to. She let this all rest within her, in her inner place of peace.

One day, on a routine follow-up visit, she was told that her chest X ray showed spots on her lung that could be lung metastasis. The darkness returned. But now she was armed by her new inner strength. This time, the depression somehow eluded her. She left the doctor's office, and as she was awaiting the films, she went directly to the arboretum nearby and looked at magnolias. She remarked that each flower was different. She said that each had its own beauty, its own shape and color, its own smell. She was taken by the differences, by the incredible sensuality, by the power of the moment. In a mysterious way, she had become the flower. From within the darkness she had found a very bright light. Her deep interest in the essence of the flower garden from far within her had taken her totally into the moment, had taken her to herself. She had let her creative passion and artistic way of seeing take her to that place, and the only point was being there. Now the flower was becoming a metaphor for her new life. As she followed her passion, she made her whole life her garden, with her family a part of it.

Nancy talked to Gina Halpern, a friend of hers who was a healing artist. Gina offered to paint a watercolor that would contain Nancy's own imagery. As the artist, Gina would paint what Nancy perceived; she would in a sense become her hands. At this point, Nancy was ill with chemotherapy, and this was easier than learning to paint by herself. Gina came over to Nancy's home and brought watercolors and large sheets of paper. They went into Nancy's garden on a beautiful spring day and talked. They looked into each other's eyes, and Gina heard Nancy's story. They talked for hours, for days. Together they decided that they would paint a mandala, a circular image that was somewhat symmetrical.

Mandalas have been used throughout history for meditation and balance. Gina had painted a series of mandalas and was familiar with this form. They stood in Nancy's garden, and Nancy saw an orange day lily in bloom that spoke to her. She decided that her central image would be that flower. She called it a "seed of darkness that would turn into a flower of hope." It became her story. Around it she had Gina paint Nancy's favorite animal, the frog. For Nancy, the frog had become a symbol of rebirth and transforma-

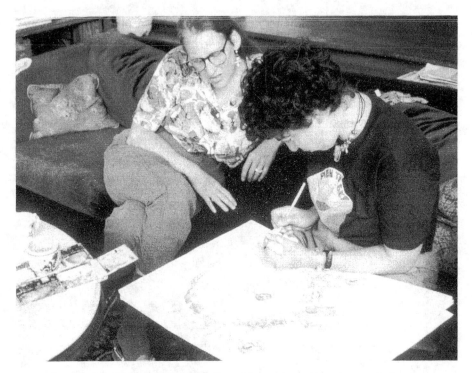

Gina Painting a Healing Mandala with Nancy. Nancy, who had breast cancer, is directing Gina to paint symbols that are part of Nancy's own healing journey. In this process, the artist is transparent and acts as Nancy's hands. This healing mandala was one of the most enjoyable and meaningful acts of healing that Nancy did for herself.

tion; it stood for Nancy's own healing, transformation, and rebirth. Gina painted the orange day lily that was blooming in Nancy's garden surrounded by the life cycle of the frog, with Nancy's frog jewelry at the bottom of the painting. Nancy chose all the colors, all the images, and told Gina where they should go. The process of working together took several days. They were both enthralled by it. The painting stood for Nancy's life. She had turned into that part of herself that was an artist. It was Nancy living most deeply in the moment. She hung the painting over her bed and looked at it each day. When she went into the hospital for a bone marrow transplant, she took it with her and hung it in the center of the wall she saw from her bed. She covered the wall with twenty feet of art. She hung paintings of flowers her friends had given her, pictures of her gardens, and all the frog sculptures she had collected and been given. This made her room an art gallery, an artist's studio, an altar, her own personal space. In the background she always played tapes of music she loved, for as she became ill she had started gardening to music and listening to music at night as she slept.

As Nancy battled breast cancer, she became an even more passionate gardener. She designed an English garden that was a mandala and carefully chose shapes and colors she loved. She slowly had her friends and family build the elaborate garden as she chose each plant. She went to England and visited the gardens she had seen in her books in the hospital. In a sense, she had found her artist within and had discovered that aspect of herself that was her healer.

Nancy was Michael Samuels's wife. She died in 1993 of breast cancer after a long battle. We feel she is very much with us in our work and in this book. She was our teacher in many ways, which is why we start this book with her story. Not all people who use art to heal can cure their illness, especially if it is a severe, life-threatening condition. Nancy had an extremely aggressive form of breast cancer. But many people with cancer and AIDS are living years longer as healing artists. We believe that many people have cured themselves of cancer, AIDS, and depression with the help of healing art. We will tell their stories throughout this book. The well-known dancer Anna Halprin healed herself of cancer with dance, and many of the patients we have worked with are now cancer free with the help of art and writing. Some people, like Nancy, heal their whole life and live every moment to the fullest. Though not everyone can be cured, their creativity can be a bridge from fear to beauty.

ART AS THE BRIDGE

How did Nancy move from the space of a woman who was ill, afraid, and depressed to the place where she experienced her life as extraordinary? Art and healing was her bridge from ordinary reality to the place where she was an artist. It became the most sacred dimension of her life in an uncanny and unacknowledged way. In some sense, she knew it was the right place to go.

It is this movement that is so precious—that is what this book is about. *Creative Healing* will connect you with others, connect you to yourself, and help you to discover the joys of being an artist.

Being creative is as simple as seeing through your eyes the beauty, mystery, and artistic quality of life. Your art, whatever form it takes, is your vehicle to go there. With Nancy it was gardening, but it was also more than that. Her garden was her art. The seeing, the choice of plants and colors, and the shapes of the paths were all her art. When she saw the magnolia flower, she was transported to another reality and her ordinary life was transcended. She saw the shapes, light, and beauty and was transported into them, away from her illness. Her music and Gina as a healing artist helped her go into this place. If you are ill or a person who wants to use art to heal others, this book will bring you into that world. It will help you heal yourself; it will help you be a healing artist.

Who is this book for? It is for the woman with breast cancer who has always wanted to be a landscape gardener, painter, or musician. It is for the man with AIDS who has always wanted to write poems or dance; the woman with asthma who does not know what she can do to breathe better but knows conventional medicine is not the only answer. It is for the woman getting a divorce who is depressed and has always yearned to paint. It is for those who are ill and do not know what they want but know something is missing from their lives. It is for the artist who wants meaning in his or her art and the healer who wants a new way to heal. It is for anyone who wants to be in service to heal a neighborhood, or the earth. It is for people who want to know who they are, who want to be themselves fully and live in all directions. It is for anyone on a spiritual path who wants to bring spirit into his or her life. It is for all of us.

How can we understand how to use art to heal? Our intention is to tell people's stories and talk about the meanings of their experiences. It is a search that will spiral us into the inner world of individuals sharing their sacred journeys of art as a new way of healing. Art gives us the ability to journey inward to a mind-body state that is deeply healing. In our imagination, we can glimpse images that heal us. Our expressions of these images can change our bodies and our lives.

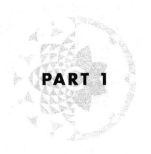

PART 1

WHAT IS
THE NEW FIELD OF
ART AND HEALING?

ONE

How Healers Use Art, Writing, Dance, and Music

Physicians and nurses are discovering that art, music, dance, and poetry have profound healing effects on their patients. Hospitals all over the world are incorporating music and art into patient care. The most sophisticated university medical centers are now creating "art in medicine" programs that invite artists and musicians to work with patients and literally change the hospital environment. These programs bring artists and musicians into the patients' rooms to make art, or have the artists perform in lobbies or atrium spaces. The patients experience the exhilaration of music or the beauty of an exhibition. They paint, play music, and dance with the artists. Art and music crack the sterile space of fear that surrounds the patients. Art opens the hospital to the joys of the human spirit. The spirit freed helps the body heal. Replacing fear with hope and darkness with light is the essence of modern body-mind-spirit medicine.

There are hundreds of art programs—both large scale and small scale—in nursing homes, hospices, community hospitals, and university medical centers. There are recreational therapy programs in drug treatment centers that use art, child life programs that use art, and community pro-

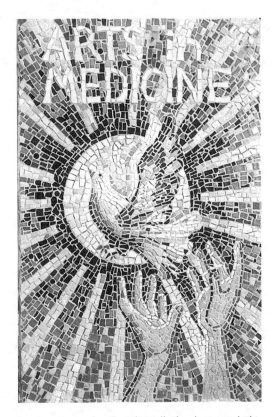

Lee Ann Stacpoole, *The Tile Wall, Shands Hospital.* This mosaic is part of the healing wall in the atrium of the hospital. Under this mosaic is written, "Since 1991, Arts In Medicine (AIM) has been exploring the many links between the creative arts and the healing arts at Shands Hospital at the University of Florida. Among us are painters and potters, singers and dancers, poets and clowns. We invite you to take ART along on your own healing journey." Each patient who comes into the hospital is given this welcome by the healing artists.

grams that use art. These invaluable grassroots programs are transforming medicine all over the world. Our intention is to illuminate these programs so that they can be recognized as the jewels they are. It is our hope that they will be integrated as part of the primary health-care model, and not segregated to the side as recreation or entertainment

We also want to acknowledge the caregivers who use art or music as part of their practice. If a nurse or other caregiver sings to a patient as part of a bath, we want the singing to be seen as just as important as the bathing, as a primary part of health care. We invite all the people associated with such programs to see themselves as critical to health care and to take seriously the making of art in a health-care setting. The artist brings spirit and hope to their hospital environment.

THE NEW FIELD OF ART AND HEALING

Art and healing is quickly becoming a new field in the world of healing and the world of making art. Art and healing has brought the creative arts, including painting, sculpture, music, dance, storytelling, and poetry, into clinical health-care settings. In art and healing, the creative arts are used for their own healing power rather than for interpretation or therapy. This new innovative approach is being integrated into the patient's health care in many settings, including bone marrow transplant units, adolescent diabetes units, adult oncology units, and outpatient cancer units. By opening the scientific paradigm of the medical center worldview, art and healing will revolutionize preconceived conventions of health care. It is a return to the illumination of beauty inherent in our humanness. Healing art is the new alternative medical therapy. It will become the next movement in holistic medicine, and each person who is ill can practice it themselves now with this book.

What has caused the growth of art and healing worldwide? Healing art is being born as we speak. The concept is catching fire, is awakening in people's spirits. The idea is being born anew. It is being born in two worlds simultaneously. In the world of art, artists, musicians, and dancers are realizing that their imagery has meaning. They are understanding that their imagery heals them, others, their neighborhood, or the earth. It is coming as a flash, an awakening. When artists make a healing image they feel such energy around them that they cannot help making more. Their lives are changed, their world is changed. The second vision comes from the world of the healer. Art in the hospital, or art at the bedside with a person who is ill, is an electrifying experience. It becomes the doorway for the spirit. It becomes the vehicle for the opening of the heart. It is integral to healing.

How does this rebirth of art and healing manifest itself in the outer world? First, now there are artists, musicians, and dancers making healing art purposely. A large body of work of this type of art is accumulating. This art heals by freeing the artists' own healing energy and resonating their body, mind, and spirit. Next, the artist can make a piece of art to heal another person. The artist can do it for specifically one person or for a group of people. This is transpersonal healing. It connects one to another; it is an art of interconnection. The third type of art heals the world. The artist makes a piece that works with the energy of a whole system, whether it be a neighborhood, an ecosystem, or the planet itself. This art can be ceremonial, environmental, performance, or static. It involves the community. It involves energy and movement. It is truly shamanic; it balances the world.

When patients make art to heal, with or without a guide, or when patients use art in their healing, we have the second broad category of healing art. Art at the bedside, art workshops for patients, art therapy, art exhibitions at hospitals, and environments in healing centers all represent this type. Again the way this art heals is the same. It does not matter whether healing art is made by an artist or a patient. It heals by making it and freeing the patient's own energy, viewing it and letting the energy be freed or participating in a ritual where the energy is freed.

ART PROGRAMS IN HOSPITALS

Initially, hospital art programs dealt with hanging art on the hospital walls and were based on the traditional model of an art gallery. When art is hung in a long, sterile hallway or sculpture is displayed in a bare lobby, the hospital is a much healthier place for everyone. These rich art programs helped transform the medical center or hospital into a place of beauty and helped relax the patients and staff. Walking down the halls past paintings of beautiful landscapes or dancing figures makes you feel completely different. You concentrate on beauty, color, and movement, you read the artist's statements, and you are taken elsewhere. Large medical centers began to have major art exhibitions, sometimes many at once, which greatly helped to humanize the center and made it feel more caring and comfortable for both patients and staff. This work was significant because it created an awareness of the hospital as an appropriate environment for art, an environment where beauty promoted healing.

Art was brought into some of the hospitals to be intentionally relaxing and healing as well as aesthetically pleasing. At the same time, the programs that had brought in art to humanize the medical center realized that the architecture of the buildings could be healing in itself. The centers started to incorporate gardens that included natural elements such as water and rocks. They built meditation rooms, chapels, and altars. Whole centers were built to communicate a sense of beauty and healing. For example, the Bailey Boushay House for AIDS patients, in Seattle, had art on almost every wall and altars in each patient's room.

Exhibitions in art museums, like the Bolinas Museum exhibition curated by Linda Samuels of the Art As A Healing Force program and the *Body and Soul* exhibition in the Decordaba Museum, also made people aware of the power of art to heal. As art programs grew in hospitals, the Society of Arts in Healthcare was formed to link the programs and help the work grow. Currently its membership includes artists, hospital art administrators, designers, physicians, nurses, and others interested in healing art. The Society of Arts in Healthcare holds annual conferences, sponsors art exhibitions, and networks people in the field.

This movement of art in hospitals has been a significant doorway to changing the way art is thought about by health-care professionals. Programs started to humanize the hospital environments by hanging art on the walls evolved to sponsoring performances or concerts in atrium spaces. Here, performers would play music or dance in the hospital lobby as they would in a concert hall. The hospital community was still the viewer in these situations rather than a participant, but performances have a deep impact on the hospital environment. When you walk through a lobby and a grand piano is being played, your entrance to the hospital has been completely changed. The music produces a soft, relaxed place where people are more meditative and open to healing.

Increasingly, artists who have experienced art as a way of healing are participating in the programs. The art hanging in the hospital setting is now more likely to be consciously related to healing than it is to aesthetics. Hollis Sigler, a painter who lives with breast cancer, has put together an exhibition of art dealing with breast cancer. The Society of Arts in Healthcare has sent her exhibition to hundreds of hospitals nationwide. Her work is profoundly moving to cancer patients and their families and to the hospital staffs. People who have seen the show have said that the hospital seemed more sensitive to their feelings, more caring. Art makes the medical center a place with a heart.

The artists participating in these programs are now much more likely to be people with health problems or people who have an understanding and passion for art as a way of healing. For the artists who are using art to heal themselves, art becomes a way of knowing about their illness. Instead of defining themselves in terms of their illness, these artists define themselves in terms of their creativity.

ART AT THE BEDSIDE

Concurrent with hospital programs that focused on art on the walls and artists in performance were programs started to focus on art at the bedside. Arts In Medicine (AIM) at the University of Florida, Gainesville, cofounded by coauthor Mary Rockwood Lane, has had more than two hundred artists working in fifteen units and puts on more than a hundred art and healing events a month. We will tell its story in detail below. In another program, Art for Recovery, painter Cindy Perliss was asked by an oncologist to work with cancer and AIDS patients. She established Art for Recovery at the University of California, San Francisco, and has been a bedside artist since 1988. Her program now also involves schoolchildren, a breast cancer quilt project, local exhibitions of patient art, and an internship program. Initially she was alone, but now a musician and other artists have joined in her work. Her program has changed the experience of many very ill patients in a magnificent way. For several years she has worked intimately with patients who are often near death. Her art is deeply spiritual, and she often forms a close relationship with her patients.

The patients' artwork is often one of the most important things in their lives. It expresses both pain and hope, and it is often their last memorial. One of her AIDS patients became such a skilled artist while in the hospital that he had an exhibition in a gallery before he died. As he created more and more paintings, he became well known in the AIDS ward as an artist, and his image was forever changed—in his eyes and in the eyes of the staff. He went from being depressed and passive to being involved in life and a goodwill ambassador representing all AIDS patients by sharing his images of the AIDS experience. His artwork was deeply moving to everyone. He attended the show and, although he was close to death, he was empowered and at peace. As he approached death, he went from hostility and loneliness to extraordinary creativity. Such an attitude change affects quality of life dramatically and may lengthen life.

Therese Schroeder-Shaker in Montana has a group of harpists who visit patients of all ages who are dying. They are called by the patients' families and it has become one of the most requested medical services in the area. She has attended more than five hundred deaths, and there are now thirty harpists playing seven days a week in Missoula. She reports that her patients have less pain and are deeply at peace, the families are relaxed, and the entire experience of dying is transformed. Her project is currently being implemented on a larger scale to reach families nationwide. In the Cleveland Rainbow Babies Hospital, Deforia Lane has set up a program to work with music and children. Many more beautiful programs across the nation are not publicized past their own community; we honor these programs, too.

This movement to integrate art in hospital settings was paralleled in the art world. Feminist artists and African American artists increasingly made art about the women's experience and celebrating the power of the goddess to heal and nourish women. Writers would come together to read poetry and journals to heal; dancers would do performances about AIDS and other illnesses. The theater world mounted plays about AIDS and healing. A common theme in all the arts was a recognition of how artists could use art to heal themselves. Keith Smith, a painter, did a magnificent book about his wife's death from

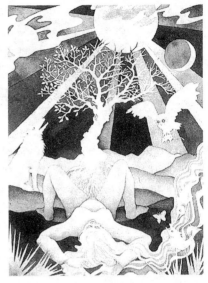

Keith Smith, *Mourning Sickness*. Keith was a professional artist and art professor in New Jersey who started to make healing art when his wife was stricken with cancer. He became a master healing artist and wrote *Mourning Sickness*, which includes illustrations and poetry about dealing with grief. Keith writes,

Mourning Sickness
growth and change
dance this dance
with
loss and pain
see the furred petaled and winged world
eating destroying being born and unfurled
searing fearful horrific and blind
peaceful potent serene and sublime
testing testing
are you prepared to conceive
to deal with
what is dealt
from the magician's sleeve
you are pregnant with God
you are great with soul
giving birth to yourself
is life's greatest goal
do not be still born again

cancer called *Mourning Sickness,* which showed all of us how poetry and art are related to healing. So an awareness of art as healing spread in the art world as well as in the hospital programs.

Networking in this area became a cultural phenomenon. In Vermont, a state arts initiative brought together all the people in the community who were interested in art and healing. People came out from isolation and joined in the effort to set up healing art as a statewide program and to help it flourish in health facilities all over northern New England. The people who joined together were as varied as the field. The regional meeting included an artist dealing with child abuse; artists running programs in nursing homes; Virginia Soffa, a woman who had had breast cancer and had set up a Breast Cancer Action slide library; and Naj Wycoff, a professor at Dartmouth working with art and medicine with medical students. They all joined to implement arts and healing in their area. When a call went out, this diverse group came together and art became an intentional healing force.

A second conference in Vermont encouraged the local university hospital to look at ways to integrate these valuable community resources into mainstream medicine. And it encouraged the community at large to look for innovative ways to integrate the arts in healing. Among conference attendees were government officials, including the state senator. It brought together leaders from volunteer agencies, funding agencies, and health organizations. A statewide arts initiative validated what people were doing on a grassroots level and helped implement projects. At the meeting, one artist suggested painting the ceiling tiles so patients lying on their backs on gurneys could see art above them as they were taken to be X-rayed or back to their rooms. The "healing ceiling" at Shands Hospital, Gainesville, which now has thousands of square feet of painted tiles, came out of that meeting. In Rhode Island, artists gathered to see how programs could grow in their state. They held a conference, sponsored several exhibitions of healing art, and organized lectures. The mayor of Providence even declared a Healing Art Week and opened the exhibition with a speech on art and healing, including references to shamanism and art. Artists are joining together, manifesting their passion for art and healing, in programs all over the country. This work is just beginning.

INTERNATIONAL PROGRAMS

There are wonderful art in medicine programs all over the world. There are rich programs in England and Australia, in Japan and France. In Australia, in a children's hospital, one artist did a mural painting with aboriginal dream-time themes. The children and their families from the hospital and the community participated, painting local animals down a long corridor. The mural was so successful that they did a second mural. It completely changed the children's wards, turning them into places of play and connection with nature.

In England, there are numerous programs of art and healing. Many of the artists in England are salaried, and the programs are deeply integrated into British health care. The programs include beautiful hospital buildings filled with sculpture and art and "art at the bedside" programs. Queen Elizabeth Hospital has a huge stained-glass window in the entry. Bristol Hospital has a touchable wall made of local clay.

In Vancouver, a conference is held to get the artists together and introduce them to health-care providers, including the therapists from the art therapy program. A pediatrician there has hung art around the beds of premature babies. The photographs of the babies' homes humanize the neonatal unit, encouraging the staff to treat the babies more like individuals. It is a good example of how art can change the care given by physicians and nurses by making the staff see the patients as more three-dimensional. When a premature baby is seen as a member of a family, the institution's whole level of care changes.

MAJOR PROGRAMS WITH NATIONAL VISIBILITY

There are hundreds of art and medicine programs across the United States, in hospitals, nursing homes, and other health-care facilities. Several of these programs have developed and grown and are now well known in the field of art and healing. An example of a successful program can be found at Boston Children's Hospital, which is filled with color and art to help the children feel at home. A program there funded by Very Special Arts makes it possible for Harvard Medical School students to participate in making art with children. The medical students work with inpatients and outpatients as an elective in their junior year. They make fun name tags in the waiting areas, and the children wear them and even give them to their doctors. Cumberland Memorial Hospital in Ohio has an entranceway where people come in under a star called Astra, a symbol of hope and endurance. The next thing patients see is a healing quilt made by a fiber artist in collaboration with the hospital staff. Poems hang on pillars in the lobby, and a healing garden serves as an oasis for everyone in the hospital.

Hospital Audiences Incorporated (HAI) in New York City concentrates on bringing patients from hospital residences, nursing homes, and day programs to community arts performances and activities. This "arts workshop" program brings professional artists to work with mentally ill adults in residences and treatment programs throughout the city. Talented artists have been discovered through this program and are currently represented by the Louise Ross Gallery. They have a special bus designed to carry patients in beds and wheelchairs to art performances all over the city. Theaters with empty seats call HAI and invite patients to performances. Lombardi Cancer Center in Georgetown, Maryland, commissioned area artists to create a painting of the Potomac River called the *River of Healing*. The painting was enlarged to two stories high, cut up, and made into waves. At the National Institutes of Health, in Washington, D.C., a changing gallery in the waiting room showcases works by local area artists. It features a bronze sculpture called *Healing Waters* that symbolizes the care of the medical center for its patients. At Mid Columbia Medical Center in Dales, Oregon, an artist has created kaleidoscopes from MRI images. This hospital has a magnificent three-story-high waterfall with rocks that fills the lobby and extends up into each floor. The sound of water is always heard in the whole hospital. The hospital is on the Columbia River, so the water sound reminds them of the river and makes the patients feel deeply at home.

San Diego Children's Hospital is full of wonderful art designed by Annette Ridenour for children, their families, and staff. There is so much art in San Diego Children's that it feels more like a children's museum. It has interactive works that engage the children and their families in waiting rooms. The art contains messages of hope, wholeness, and wellness. St.

Joseph's Hospital in Phoenix, Arizona, has display cases that show the pride the community has taken in the hospital and how it was made by the community. At Paradise Medical Center in San Diego, artworks by local artists celebrate multicultural holidays, family, multicultural healing rituals, and our relationship with nature. Local artists were brought in to make art that was sacred and that would help link the patients to the traditional healing patterns of their culture. Hasbro Children's Hospital in Providence, Rhode Island, has a "museum on rounds" program, where pieces of art from the Rhode Island School of Design Museum are shown to children. The children then make their own art based on the pieces from the collection, working in groups in family rooms or one-on-one at the bedside. This hospital is filled with art, murals, fountains, gardens, and sculpture and even has a zoo. Marin General Hospital in Greenbrae, California, has a healing garden by Topher Delaney that features healing plants used for treating cancer. It is part of a meditation garden. The hospital also has photo transparencies above the X-ray machines so patients lying down can see nature scenes.

The rich program at Duke University started twenty years ago with performances in the atrium. Now performers come to the patients' rooms to play music. The program is run by Janice Palmer, who has pioneered this work and has been a major force in art and healing for twenty years. Duke also has a play-reading group that meets every Friday. Called the Osler Literary Round Table, it encourages staff and patients to read poetry and short stories. At Duke, artwork was put in the patients' rooms before it was put anywhere else in the hospital. In the obstetrics ward, there are ninety-eight quilts by local quilters. The artwork in the pediatric unit is all at a child's eye level. In the eye center, there is touchable art for sight-impaired people, including a touchable gallery in the entry that's open all day. There is also a fragrance garden designed as a sun dial to follow the seasonal lines of the sun. There are birdhouse villages made by local artisans that the children can see and feel at home with. These programs give you some idea of the scope of "art in healing" programs in hospitals. We hope they encourage you to form your own ideas and programs as you become a healing artist.

Mary Tells the Story of the Arts In Medicine Program at the University of Florida

Every program starts with someone's individual story and personal initiative. I believe that everyone who has passion to create something can do it. There are always obstacles and hurdles to overcome, but they are just part of the process. My story starts with my own personal experience of art as healing. It is grounded in my experience of how profoundly art transformed my life. It's the truth that art healed my life. This connection to art became my lifework. I felt deeply committed to the creative process. Wherever it took me, I would go. I followed my passion to be an artist. I realized that being a studio artist was not enough for me. I loved it, but I needed to find a way for my art to be in service to people.

Since I was a nurse and art had healed me, I hoped to bring art into the health-care system. This was my opportunity to help others help themselves. No one had ever told me I could take my illness and use it constructively to help myself. Everywhere I looked it seemed that I had been in relationship with a form of healing that was disjointed from my life. It did not support me in the way I needed it to. It wasn't until I threw myself into my creative work that I felt a powerful healing effect. I needed to put my whole life into something powerful. I needed my whole life enmeshed in it because that was how I was involved with my sickness. Creative healing transformed my life. I pulled it out of myself and healed myself. It was not fragmented, one hour twice a week. My illness was so overwhelming I needed to live my healing all the time, not just in visits to a therapist. What was going to heal me was a relationship with myself that was fundamentally different from any I had had before. I could always be there for myself.

I remember the day that Lee Ann Stacpoole and I were in the studio, painting. I told her I had found this book, *The Reenchantment of Art* by Susie Gablik, and read about artists healing themselves, others, and the earth. It challenged me as an artist. It said, make your art meaningful in the world. You will have to make art meaningful again, you will have to make it part of service your-self. I knew that no one would suggest that I bring art into the hospital; I needed to do it on my own. We live in a world where we are in touch with others. We live in community, and so we have to go to others to get things done. I believed that we could reach out and help others.

I heard *The Reenchantment of Art* as a call to artists who were willing to integrate their art in new uncharted territories, to make it different from before. I came to it from an artist's perspective. I waited. I had to be patient. I had to wait and be awake for an opportunity to present itself. I could see that. Then one day I got a newsletter from a physician in a local hospital about his ideas about arts in medicine and about how to bring art into the med-ical school. I saw that this was someone with ideas similar to mine. I realized that at this point in the process, I needed to form a partnership. I had visions of artists coming into the hospital to work with patients; he had visions of artists in the medical school working with students. We could bring a combination of both visions to life. I met with him. We talked. I thought about how it could happen. I talked to other people, to other physi-cians, and I began to sense what I could do. I decided I wanted to start an "artist in residence" program. I would find an artist who would bring the art into the hospital in a creative and innovative way. I would bring the artist to where there was the most illness, creating a window of opportunity in which people could inte-grate the arts and become involved in their own creativity. The assumption was that everyone was an artist.

We got a small grant from the Children's Miracle Network and the first artist-in-residence was my best friend, Lee Ann Stacpoole, the woman who had helped me to paint when I was ill. I asked her to come into the hospital as a volunteer. We started in the bone marrow transplant unit because the physician with whom I formed the partnership, Dr. John Graham-Pole, was a pedi-atric oncologist in charge of that unit. I thought I would do this for years, five at least. I then went to the college of nursing to earn a Ph.D. so I could get involved in a university program that would be the backbone for my art and healing and to create an educational process that would ground me and keep me focused. I was committed to it, and I knew it was my lifework. Lee Ann and I started as two "ordinary housewives," two artists in the studio, and we created another partnership. I realized that the commitment was something we would do for a long time. Our logo, "passion with patience," was born in the midst of the beginning fires of energy and passion with the velocity of the universe being born. We had to stay grounded so that we would do it, and so it would mature. We needed patience, because otherwise it would burn itself out. You need to maintain passion and let things grow naturally, and you also need enough time for a doorway to open and allow people space to become who they are.

The second artist-in-residence was Mary Lisa Katakis, a painter who also was a T-shirt artist. She was asked to come into the program by one of the nurses we worked with. As the program grew, we were overwhelmed by people's interest. I told Mary Lisa that we would be here for the long run. Knowing that you are committed to the program in spite of the low salary and being able to stay focused and grounded in what you can accomplish is essential. When you stay focused, you accomplish an incredible amount. When you start a program, you realize that artists are filled with generosity, abundance, and creativity. They are exploding with possibilities. Their capability for expression is immense. A critical mass of artists is like a wellspring from the earth.

I said that we would find an appropriate venue for each artist who comes to us, whether that would be performing in the atrium, working with patients on a unit, making puppets, being a student volunteer, or implementing a two-year tile project. We can find endless opportunities. The most essential component is someone who is willing to harness the creative energy, the chaos, to keep people focused on their own creativity, to honor them and see them—a person who can let each artist articulate his or her own vision and dream. When you believe in the artists, they believe in themselves and in the inherent creativity of the patients and staff. We had a passionate intention to heal.

It began completely with volunteers. With our grant we bought art supplies and set up a studio space in the bone marrow transplant ward where artists could meet. Then we started networking. For the first two years we did nothing but network. Everybody was invited to the meetings then. We were networking monthly. We would present our vision to others in the medical school and the veterinary school, to art educators, to social workers, to nursing supervisors. We talked with everyone. We told everyone what our vision was.

AIM now has had over two hundred artists in fifteen units. It has evolved to become a part of the hospital structure. AIM currently consists of artists-in-residence who do a variety of creative projects. There are now a musician, a visual artist, a dancer, and a storyteller in residence. There are also many artists who come in one or two days a week and work in the program for months or years. The artists play music, dance, draw, and sculpt. They write poetry, tell stories, and even dress as clowns. Patients watch, tell the artists what they want them to do, or make art alongside the artists. Performances of music, dance, poetry, or theater are put on in the hospital lobby. Patients are brought from their rooms, families and staff stop as they go to lunch, the music drifts through the sterile corridors and draws more people toward its transformational power. Patients and staff alike leave relaxed and uplifted; they are changed and healed.

The musician-in-residence, Cathy DeWitt, plays her piano in the atrium in a weekly series. She also works one-on-one with patients. The musicians serenade like strolling musicians or they play personally for a patient in his or her own room. Cathy and the other musicians have an active music program, which has had a profound and enriching effect on the hospital environment. The musician has become an important part of the healing process. Of all artists, musicians are most easily integrated in a variety of settings. Musicians can perform or they can serenade families in support groups on individual units. They bring in their own music as well as instruments so that the process can become interactive. For example, they encourage a young patient who knows the guitar to play. They jam, they create situations to jam on wards. Family and staff can join in. They create songs and sing-alongs. Cathy also plays and brings community musicians who are friends

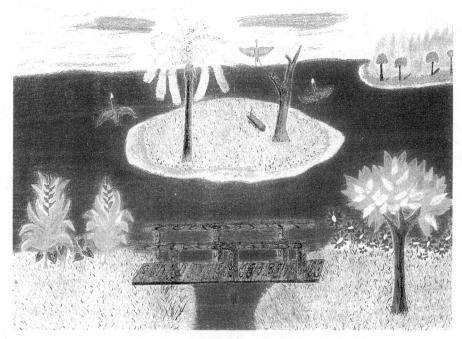

William Clem, *Untitled.* When William was having a bone marrow transplant for cancer, he painted a series of seventy-two watercolors to help heal himself. William says, "In the midst of a life-threatening illness and all the negativity and fear that accompany it, I found art again. I also found that my style of drawing helps me focus on the beautiful things life has to offer. The pictures and the process of drawing the pictures help me face the possibility of my death with strength and also to face myself in a positive light. The Arts In Medicine program (at Shands Hospital) helped and is still helping me to share my feelings and experiences through my art. I will always be grateful and remember Shands and all the loving and caring people who helped me fight for my life. I will never forget!"

into the atrium for concerts. People who walk into the lobby to be treated or to visit can hear live music. It reaches patients, staff, the entire hospital community. We also have a harpist and flutists. They have found that drumming is hard for very sick patients, who are often oversensitized, so they concentrate on softer music. There is even a musician who plays the accordion, and a strolling barbershop quartet that has been a tremendous success. We have found the strolling musicians are ancient healers.

The dancer-in-residence, Jill Henderson, created a "dance for life" program. Jill works one-on-one and does support groups primarily on the pediatric bone marrow transplant ward. She forms long-term relationships with the children. She follows the child and begins to create a dance for his or her life. She introduces herself as a dancer and invites the children to dance with her or asks if she can dance for them. She brings in music. When the music starts, she moves the children. She moves with them, she opens up the possibility for children to become the directors of their own dances. The dancer-in-residence brings in other dancers; Jill has twelve student dancers and they are all dancing with children in thirteen different units.

The visual artists program includes the tile wall project, the healing ceiling (which involves painting foam ceiling tiles so patients see healing paintings made by children, staff, and family when they look up). There are murals, dream catchers, medicine wheels, origami paper cranes—each one a prayer—and T-shirts painted one-on-one. A patient often completes a huge number of paintings. A bone marrow transplant patient named William Clem painted a series of watercolors during his treatment. Visual-artists-in-residence also use Fimo clay to make objects, flowers, animals, necklaces, and ornaments. They use clay with patients, with family, and in support groups. Photographers give people cameras to take pictures and encourage them to write stories. Artists go into patients' rooms and people often tell them what to paint, saying that they want butterflies or ten daisies. People know very specifically what they want. The visual artists also make hats, teddy bears, quilts, and presents for holidays.

There are storytellers-in-residence who read and tell stories. They publish *Zine* magazine, an underground newspaper in which children tell their own stories of being in the hospital. They share their perspective of being ill. The magazine is circulated among the children so they can read stories of children who are hospitalized on a different floor. It creates an underground communication network where children can feel that they are part of a community. The storytellers incorporate games, puppets, musicians, songs, dance, and other arts. There is also a theater program in AIM. The Playback Theater is a troupe that sits with patients and enacts patients' stories. A professor from the theater department of the University of Florida does theater and theater games with psychiatric adolescent patients. The artists work on a variety of units, including such units as the bone marrow transplant, pediatric intensive care, diabetic adolescent, psychiatry, autistic children, general oncology, medicine, gynecology, surgery, mother-baby, and even the dental waiting room. Artists will go into any clinical area that is accessible to them or that they are asked to work in. Artists get patient referrals and go into new units, such as the sickle cell unit, to do imagery. The daily work changes and evolves depending on the artists who are there and the caregivers who work with them. One of the most exciting parts of the program now is its flexibility, creativity, inclusiveness, and speed of implementing new ideas. If you walk into the program and look around and think of a unique way to work as an artist with patients, you can put your ideas into action almost instantly.

Patients at the University of Florida who are visited by Arts In Medicine artists say their whole experience of being ill is changed forever. They are more hopeful and happier, feel better, and have less pain. This process takes place whether the patients or their families watch the artists or make art themselves. Even if they just watch, they still are an audience participating with their hearts. If they are too sick to paint, they can see themselves being painted or tell the artist what to draw. They often ask for a favorite scene, an animal, their child. Studies in progress now have shown that patients who feel better about themselves and are more hopeful live longer with cancer. People who are in touch with their own creativity are in a state of joy and hope.

There are many beautiful projects that artists do in Arts In Medicine. The healing tile wall is the illumination of embodied moments of making art. In a studio at the hospital, the child with cancer, the parents, the staff—anyone who wanted to—could come in and paint a tile. Each tile told a story. When we first set up the studio and got the materials together, we felt touched by a certain luminosity. It was like seeing the light on the leaves. What we saw in each tile was an illumination of a precious moment in which someone went deeply into his or her own soul to make art. The project taught us that making art is transitory; it happens in a moment.

The first person who came into the room was a mother with a child receiving chemotherapy. The child was playful, but the mother shook her head and said, "I can't paint." Lee Ann said, "I can help you." The materials were all there, but the mother sat for a long time thinking. She asked quietly, "Would you mind if I painted a tile for my little daughter who died in September?" For the first time, the woman felt she had been given the opportunity to make something that would remain. For the next hour, she almost meditatively painted her lost child's name in different colors and wrote "I love you" and the date that her child had died. The mother became absorbed and transfixed in a busy hospital, while her other child was getting treatment. She quickly went to a very private place within that was all about her painting. Time was suspended as the mother became very focused in making this tile. It was obvious that this was important to her. She asked, "So, are you going to put this tile in a wall so I can come back and see it?" Lee Ann explained that there would be a healing wall.

A teenager painted himself on a tile as a brave hero and showed the tile to a little child with the same leukemia as his who was about to have the same bone marrow transplant. They then made a tile together that portrayed both of them holding hands. The tile was called *Two Brave Men*. Tile painting is so easy it could be done by everyone who walked in, without any training. The tile wall, which consists of more than a thousand tiles, now hangs in the hospital atrium for patients, family, and staff to see each time they come to the hospital. Beautiful mosaics surround the tile wall, capturing the themes and some of the recurring images seen in the individual tiles. The wall is lovingly crafted to complement the art the patients made. Lee Ann created the mosaic after her son was born with Downs syndrome. The artwork gave her a community and a project when she needed support.

These are the kinds of projects artists do. They are simply community artists who have come in, negotiated with staff and caregivers, made a commitment of their time, brought in the supplies, and been there for the patients. The projects go on for a week, a year, or two years, but each one is about an artist who has negotiated with a physician or nurse running a unit to set up a studio and work with their patients. It happens because someone goes in and makes it happen. Artists cannot wait to be asked; they go in as guests. They need to be receptive and totally honor what is going on in the setting. Here they did it by simply creating a studio space where the patients could work. The patients were getting all-day chemotherapy. The patients would come in for months at a time; they were there.

The AIM program is a shared vision between artists and caregivers. At the University of Florida, it is deeply tied to nursing care. The nurses are vital participants in the program. Every artist who comes on a unit is in communication with a nurse. Physicians and nurses write prescriptions for art just as they would for a drug or other intervention. As the focus of health care changes from cure to care, nursing is providing leadership and a vision for others. AIM has become a clinical model for the nursing practice to integrate the "arts in care" practice and for nurses to choose creative art interventions in responding to patients' needs. We advocate the presence of artists inside the hospital to teach and facilitate how the arts can be implemented right at the patient's bedside as the patient gets chemotherapy and other medical treatments. The nurse is the facilitator and an advocate for the patient's voice in this process. The nurse has a deep knowledge of how this can happen and the power to manifest it for the patient's care.

HOW ART AND HEALING DIFFERS FROM ART THERAPY

Art therapy has been a major force in art and healing for many years. Art therapy, music therapy, dance therapy, poetry therapy, and writing therapy are all mature fields with wonderful creative practitioners who meld the arts with psychotherapy to heal. Expressive arts therapy uses art as a creative force to work with patients in ways as varied as the practitioners who grace this beautiful field.

Traditionally, art therapy involved people who used art to diagnose, analyze, and interpret an individual's psychological processes. The artwork was used in art therapy to try to resolve patients' problems and help them gain insight through the imagery they drew. Through art, the person's inner process would be revealed and become accessible to the patient and the therapist. It was a powerful healing technique that used all the art forms to deal with grief, anger, and emotional and psychological illnesses.

The model of art therapy is often different from art and healing as portrayed in this book because art therapy is formally integrated into a diagnosis and treatment model that includes medical classification, taxonomy, and reimbursement. It also involves a specific training, a degree, a license, and a defined role in a medical setting. Unfortunately, it has been difficult to integrate fully into the mainstream medical model due to reimbursement systems, though in some settings it works well.

The focus of art therapy is on interpretation and analysis. The people involved are primarily therapists, not artists. Using traditional psychological models, the therapist helps the patient deal with areas of conflict. More art is made as the process continues, which reflects the healing and helps it occur. In expressive arts therapy, the therapist helps the patient make art, dance, paint, or write. The work of art is believed to help the patient deal with the areas of conflict, and the therapist helps by interpreting the artwork created.

At this point in time, art therapy and expressive arts therapy are much broader than they used to be and are extremely creative and innovative. They both run the spectrum from psychotherapy to art and healing, and each therapist has his or her own way of working that varies from traditional psychotherapy to creating healing art. Right now there are people in art therapy and in expressive arts therapy who do art in healing the same way we discuss in this book and others who are traditional therapists. But currently there are basic differences in the approaches of the fields that make them separate and unique. Each has its own power, and each is right for some patients and some artists. Art and healing provides a new alternative to artists who want to work with patients and not do therapy or be licensed, and a new alternative to patients who want to make art and not be in any kind of therapy. It is the right path for many artists and patients.

The basic belief of art and healing is that an artist can be with another person just to make art, and that that process is healing in itself. There is no diagnosis, classification, treatment, or outcome measurement other than the patient's experience of the process as being meaningful. Expressive arts therapy often bridges the two fields of art and healing and art therapy. It involves characteristics of both and can primarily focus on one or the other in practice. Art therapy today also can be art and healing without therapy or interpretation, or strict psychotherapy, depending on the person and the program. Also, art therapists can work in art and healing programs along with artists. Art therapy is a powerful healing technique that has contributed much to art and healing and to medicine.

Currently, we believe that there is no need for licenses to certify artists in art and healing. The only license you need to be with another human being in a time of suffering is to be human, to be present, and to have the intention to be healing. What we have found in the most powerful work is the person's intention to heal, to be a witness to the creative process, to be clear, and to allow the patient the space to be creative without imposing an opinion—without any criticism at all. The intention to heal is critical. The merging of the two people's spirits is magical. One person has the intent to be healed, one person the intention to heal. You join and create a caring encounter. Art is just the vehicle for love, for joining. The artist embraces the person's painting as the finest expression of the individual's life. It is art at its finest because it is taken as something we do together with another person in a new level of meaningfulness.

HEALING ENVIRONMENTS: CHANGING THE HOSPITAL

> The effect in sickness of beautiful objects, of a variety of objects and especially of brilliancy of color is hardly at all appreciated. I have seen in fevers (and felt, when I was a fever patient myself) that most acute suffering was produced from the patient not being able to see out of the window and the knots in the wood being the only view. I shall never forget the rapture of fever patients over a bunch of bright colored flowers. People say the effect is only on the mind. It is no such thing. The effect is on the body, too. Little as we know about the way in which we are affected by form, by color and light, we do know this: they have an actual physical effect. Variety of form and brilliancy of color in the objects presented to patients are actual means of recovery.
>
> Florence Nightingale, 1888

Since ancient times, environments have been crucial for healing. In Navaho sand paintings, an environment for healing was made that told a spiritual story from the person's culture. The patient was put right on the sand painting and was then part of the whole world of ancient spirits and was in the nonordinary space of healing. In Greece, in Delphi, the healing temples were in areas of great beauty and were sanctuaries of healing. They were located in magnificent natural sites and had sacred springs, mountains, or rivers nearby. It took a pilgrimage to get to the healing temples. They were believed to be on sacred sites where earth energies were strongest.

In modern hospitals, we realize increasingly that we need to create environments in the hospital that are healing and make a person feel cared for. When people come into buildings that are huge or out of scale, they do not feel at home. It's important to make this environment comfortable. Textures and colors communicate feelings. Traditionally, hospitals have been sterile, monumental buildings that make you feel alienated and not at home. At times they have been huge complexes, with long corridors and hidden faces. It is hard for a person to feel oriented, to feel a human presence. The lack of sensitivity to views—to what is seen out of windows—has been incredible. We believe this criticism is important. Hospital environments can be disorienting with their strange noises, and often the atmosphere seems to be in direct contradiction to healing. These buildings themselves need to be healed. The communities within hospitals need to be healed. Art is the way to heal these environments.

CREATING A HEALING ENVIRONMENT IN OUR HOMES

Last but not least, it is essential that we create a healing environment in our homes. We heal ourselves by creating and maintaining our own healing space. We can do this by creating a relationship with nature, with sunlight, and by opening up the views to the outside. It is as beautiful as bringing in flowers from the garden and letting in the sunlight. Creating a healing environment also includes the company of good friends and family and bringing in positive healing sounds of nature. Inside our homes, we can create a sacred space where we honor ourselves and our homes' physical energy. We can make our own altars. We can position artwork where we can see it when we walk around the halls. We can use paintings as windows. The artwork can change our perspective and bring into our lives colors and vibrant images that are life-enhancing. We also can create sacred time within the environment that becomes part of our lived experience of healing.

A GUIDED IMAGERY EXERCISE TO FEEL CREATIVE HEALING

You can feel healing energy and experience creative healing right now. Throughout this book we will use guided imagery as a way to go deeper into our feelings, evoking personal images and/or memories. Guided imagery is a medically proven technique for healing and an age-old technique for promoting spiritual growth. To use imagery, just relax, read the words on the page, and let your mind follow. Let your imagination take you wherever you want to go. You don't have to do anything. Just picture what comes into your mind's eye. You can let it happen while you read, or read a paragraph and then imagine it in your mind's eye. Or you can let someone read the imagery to you as you close your eyes and relax. Any way is fine. As you read this book, you will get better at doing the imagery. This first imagery exercise is just to let you feel imagery. For now, simply let the process happen and don't expect anything specific.

> Relax; let your breathing slow. Take several deep breaths. Let your abdomen rise and fall as you breathe. Now, for a moment, let your heart open. In your mind's eye, see it actually open, like a flower opening, like hands opening, like doors opening. Rest a moment and let those feelings take you deeper. Now imagine you, or a loved one, ill and in need of love. Picture them in your mind's eye. Let yourself be deeply moved by these images. Stop—rest there; feel the emotions. Let the feelings within you come out. Feel images of sadness and of love and healing. Feel the differences between the two spaces of sadness and healing. Allow your emotions to surface—open your heart; feel grief; feel love; feel healing.

> Now we will journey into art, music, and dance. We will be there for a moment. First discover your own images of the illness. See an area that is ill; see cells, or see darkness. Now feel your own artist healer arrive. Feel a presence of a loving, caring being come; feel a part of you that emerges from within to help you heal. Now, in your imagination, let yourself see a healing image

replace your image of illness. It can be a flower, a white blood cell eating a cancer cell, a rainbow, a scene in a forest, a loved one, a teacher, a spiritual leader. Let the healing forces change your image of illness. Let the white blood cell eat the cancer cell, the rainbow bring light into the darkness. Just let it happen. If you don't feel anything, just let yourself relax deeply and rest.

Now take the image of healing and make it into art. In your imagination, make a painting, a poem, a prayer, a song, a dance. Take the image of light, beauty, and healing and let it be art. Give yourself time for this to happen; let the art appear in front of your eyes. Now see how you feel—feel your body as you make the art. Feel your energy, your calmness, your concentration. Look at your transformation; feel its peace and beauty. Let images slip into your consciousness; feel the energy in lines and dots, in sounds, in movement. Now imagine that you are the healing images that you made, you are the rainbow, the light, the God you may have portrayed, the spirits you may have seen. Feel the visions as power. Let your body be a receiver for God's message.

To finish up, let any thoughts you had of illness flow out of you. Let the images of illness you have invited in to look at leave now. Let them leave until all images of illness are gone. Now let light flow in, let light come to you, over you, around you. Imagine you or your loved one are completely healed. Feel the power within you rise; feel your center strengthen. Rest in the moments between your breaths. Now open your eyes, look around you, and bring the transformative power of art, writing, music, and dance out into your life. Bring the power of your imagery back with you into your room. It will be with you always.

You can see that creative healing is not a passive art form. Healing art is not meant to be passively watched. This is about your life force. This art is made to change reality. We are on the doorstep of a great journey. Imagine where we can go. Imagine art, music, and dance in every hospital, art with anyone who is ill. Imagine lifting the spirits of someone who is very ill. Imagine being in love.

We intend this book to be a gift to you, an offering. You will find your gift in your own heart. This book is your guide, and your helper. This book will help you to see the reflection of yourself as the artist that you are. You have opened the door to allow your inner healer to speak to you through your creative process. The form of your own communication and particular expression is up to you. The form emerges from your own life force and innate creative impulse. The artist is like the lion tamer; the lion's roar is the truth. The artist holds the space for the healer to speak. The artist harnesses the forces that create and maintain the world.

We hope that this book will help you heal yourself, change your consciousness, and change your life. These "modest" goals feel real to us because of our immense passion for art and healing and because of our wonderful experiences with art and healing in our own lives, with patients in medical centers, with artists, and with environmental artists. We believe that each of us is part of the worldwide puzzle that makes up the earth, and that as we become ourselves we heal each other and the world. Welcome to *Creative Healing*. We hope it will be a wonderful journey for you, one that will free your artist and your healer and fill you with light and bring you into your own light, into your own illumination.

TWO

How Art
and Healing
Are One

The basic message of *Creative Healing* is very simple. Art heals you, art heals others, and art heals the earth. Each of us has deep within us an inner artist and an inner healer. The inner artist is the part of us that is passionately creative, that feels love, that feels connected to everything around us, that can see, that knows who we are, that is at home, and that is at peace.

The inner artist can go anywhere in the inner world. No place is closed to it. It can even go to the inner healer and merge with it and bring it out. The inner healer is the part of you that balances your body perfectly and sets your blood flow, your immune system, and your killer T cells to be in harmony. Art frees the healer within so you can heal yourself of an illness. Art frees your spirit so your mind and body are in harmony. Art frees your immune system to work at its optimum and help you heal. Art helps you conquer disease by freeing your inner healer to work at its optimum.

A "LET'S SAY" STORY

Let's say there is an aspect of you that you cannot see. And even more puzzling, it is the wisest and deepest aspect of who you are. Let's say that you are an ordinary woman or an ordinary man. You go through your daily routine—pick up your kids, run a business, do all the things you do—and still you somehow feel confused, disconnected from something deeper within you. You have a feeling that there is something missing, almost a life unlived. And then, one day, you get a diagnosis that you are ill, or find yourself in crisis. It could be any illness, or a life event that results in a deep depression. You go to all kinds of health-care providers, physicians, psychologists, and alternative healers to seek healing. You take herbs, do exercise, get body work done, and utilize many different types of therapies. They all help to differing degrees, but none of them feels like the essence of healing. Your body experiences itself as ill and you feel disconnected from it and betrayed by it. You know that deeper within your body is the source of your life, and now that you are ill you feel the need to make contact with this source. Somehow you know if

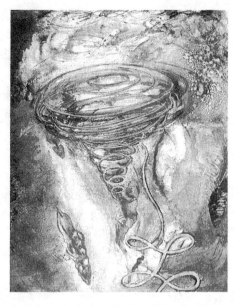

Carol Levy, *Beginnings*. Go inward on a journey to become your inner artist. Go deep into the sacred spiral. The sacred spiral comes from our most ancient memories. Carol says, "For the last twelve years I have immersed myself on a path involving the Buddhist teachings, specifically, awakening, seeing through the true nature of things, seeing the interconnectedness of things, being with what is, and lightening up. Caring for my mother for three years and being with her dying process has also been a very strong force along this path."

you can make the connection to that part of yourself it will help you heal.

Now let's say you can make art, any art, and that this process will help you find the part of yourself that will heal, the part of yourself you have been looking for. Let's say it is that simple. Let's say that all you have to do is to find the part of yourself that can say "I am an artist." All you have to do is allow yourself to be more creative, to move, sing, write, dance, and do so spontaneously, without censorship. Let's say that if you allow your creativity to be seen, it will liberate you so you can get in touch with the healer within. For example, when you paint with abandon, you find an aspect of yourself that knows the truth. You are manifesting your own creativity. This creativity is your passion; this passion is your life. Slowly, something within you starts to stir. As you realize that you are the source, you realize that you are what you need to heal.

You can picture art and healing like a hero's journey, a myth, a story, or a fairy tale. Picture yourself as a person who needs to heal your land of a great problem or evil. You travel to a foreign land you have never seen before to find helpers. You go into the forests, the mountains, the deserts, and the darkest places. You meet a person who is pure magic, a teacher, a seer. That person leads you to a secret place where the person who has the power to heal or solve the problem lives and introduces you. The healer is stuck in a cave or prison and needs to be freed. Only you can perform the feat that lets the healer out to heal the land. You throw the ring in the fire, or say a prayer, or do a dance, and the healer comes out and is free and his or her enormous power heals the land.

Of course, the meaning of this story is clear. You are the one who will be healed. The land is the inner world of your imagination. The figure who is the seer is you as the artist. The figure who is the healer is you, too. It is all you. It only seems like they are different parts. This journey will bring you to them. This journey will make the story true.

When we each find our own song, as Larry LeShan says in *Cancer as a Turning Point,* and find out what we love most, our self-healing mechanisms begin to function at their optimum. Deep within all of us is the place of perfect beauty from which we all come. It is the same place from which we are born. It is the same place to which we will return. In that place, we will find our deepest peace, our most profound memories of who we are. In our lives, this is the place of the memory of our brightest moment. It is tied to our vision of being touched, being nurtured, being loved perfectly, being in the presence of something greater than ourselves. And it is tied to our memory of our greatest sadness, of our losses, of our fears of our own death. In the center of this place of beauty is the energy that heals us. This is also the energy of our own passionate creativity.

A GUIDED IMAGERY STORY OF ART AND HEALING: THE LEGEND OF THE OLD WOMAN OF THE SPRINGS

Stories have always been used by healers. We are taught most profoundly by symbols, morals, and archetypes whose meanings sink in without our always understanding them at first. This is why fairy tales were told to children, why stories from the Bible, the Koran, or the Vedas were told to help people feel the presence of a greater power, why even older myths and legends have always been used to help people grasp the ineffable, the sacred.

Guided imagery as a mind-body therapy is also deeply relaxing and experiential. It is a basic tool in medicine, used for many illnesses. It is used in cancer clinics worldwide to help cancer patients relax and heal. Guided imagery is as simple as picturing an event or memory in your imagination. If you relax and close your eyes and picture your bedroom, you can look around in your imagination and "see" your bed, your dresser, the windows, and the color of the walls. When you use guided imagery for healing, you can picture an illness and your body's healing mechanisms. For example, you can picture cancer cells and your white blood cells eating them. We did this in the first imagery exercise in the previous chapter.

Michael has used guided imagery with cancer patients for twenty-five years, and the artists in Mary's program all use guided imagery, whether they dance, draw, or tell stories.

The legend of the old woman of the springs that we are about to tell is an ancient myth that links art and healing. It talks about how art and healing were one in a mythical time of spirits and how we are still connected to our ancestors through deep memories and our own physiology. The legend itself is as old as any story, and aspects of it appear in Native American legends, Jewish lore, Sufi myths, and African stories. The legend of the old woman of the springs is about the wellspring of creativity that is within each of us. It is about creation, connections, and our birth.

It is also a story about your being loved perfectly for who you are right now. In the legend, the old woman of the springs, who created you, loves you even if you are ill, in crisis, depressed, or lost. She loves you into the very center of your sadness, the deepest heart of your pain, the core of your anger. In a real sense, the old woman of the springs is our ancient mother. And we all have the memories of being inside our mother's body in the soft whooshing, the moving, the dimmed colors, the lub-dub of her heartbeat, the flowing sounds of her breathing. This is the first healing art, music, and dance that we recall. This ancient legend brings us there as softly as she sings. Do you hear her voice? Healing art is about going back into the place where we were loved perfectly, and where we were embraced by sound, color, and movement. It is about loving yourself for who you are right now and being seen and honored for who you are right now. In the legend, the old woman is the one who nurtures us in that way. For you, the old woman can be anyone, even an old man—gender is not important here. In this book, the love starts from inside of you.

All through this book we take the story of the old woman of the springs and expand it and use it to help you understand how art heals. Whenever we tell the story, you can rest. You don't have to think, analyze, understand, or learn anything. Each time the story is told, let it take hold of you as if it were a lullaby. Relax, have fun, be entertained. Let yourself heal.

I will tell you a story. It is a story that is older than any other. This story is deep in our memories. This story is deep in your soul. It is the story of the creation of art and healing. It always begins with the story of the old woman of the springs. She has always been seen as the weaver of our dreams, as the mother of creativity and art, as the one who could heal. Close your eyes; relax; let your breathing slow down. We will start from the ordinary, from your kitchen table, from a drive in your car, or a hospital room, from wherever you are. And we will take you deeper. We will go into our imagination on a journey.

Let us go into a mystical forest. It is a secret place. It is the place that only you can see. It is a place in your imagination. You can find it in any moment. You will find it by becoming ill, by being in a life crisis, by seeing death, by falling in love, by becoming an artist. First, imagine that you are on a path. It is a narrow path; the ground is dirt, hard enough so it is comfortable to walk on. It is the path of the creative healer. As your feet find it, you can imagine that you start to walk. Feel the hard ground—hear your footsteps fall; feel the grass on the sides of the path touch your legs. Smell the air; feel the warm soft breeze on your face. As you walk, you begin to feel different. The air itself changes. It opens and fills with light. It expands, and as it expands, you expand, too. Your eyes open wider. Your ears can hear more clearly. Your body moves by itself, and your breath is not only yours anymore.

As you go down the path, your way darkens and narrows slightly. The leaves touch your skin and the soft earth caresses your feet. The warm moist air glistens on the leaves like dewdrops and the energy within you flows outward. As you look ahead, you can see an emerald pool down a short hill. It is round and beautiful and it shines in the afternoon sun. It is at the bottom of a glade of small trees. The pool is deep blue and perfectly round and in its center is a spring that flows upward from the earth as pure clear water. You can see the bubbles coming to the surface in whirlpools; you can almost hear the bubbling as it goes on forever.

Now look upward on the ground next to the spring. Above the spring she sits, in perfect and eternal peace. She is the most beautiful creature you have ever seen. She is a woman of pure spirit. As you look at her, you can see that she changes as you see her. One moment she is the Virgin Mary looking down on you with perfect love. One moment she is your lover, looking at you with eternal desire, and in the next moment she is an old woman with a loom who weaves the silver and golden threads that make the springs and the earth itself. And then, in another moment, she is a turtle who has sat forever on the side of the spring watching all of it being born. As she sits and changes like the light, you can see that she has been there forever and has created the world. She weaves the fibers of her most beautiful dream. She weaves art and healing as one. She weaves each of us into the vision as artists, as healers. She weaves the very spirals that we travel on, and the energy that makes us fall in love. She is weaving this story as I am telling it to you. She is weaving this book as her song on earth. She is singing to us.

Now look more closely. She sits on the edge of the spring, and as she looks down inside the spring, she can see the eternal well-spring of creativity and she can see your life. She has meditated here for a million years, and she can see the water spring up from the very center of her own heart. She sees how beautiful she is, was, and will be. She sees how it always flows, and how it will flow for a million lifetimes. For each lifetime, for each of our ancestors before us from the first one, she has sat there. She has been there for all of eternity.

You can see that out of the spring comes a turquoise light. It shines on her face and on yours. You can see that she is very ancient. If you look closely you can see that a part of her is young and youthful, and a part of her is very old. Look at her hands. As she sits and you look at her hands, it is almost as if she holds a magic wand from which she is weaving a magic web. You can see that she looks deep into the springs, and from the center of the spring you can see the energy go up into her hands. She weaves a magic web for you. She catches the spring's energy and power, and weaves it into the earth. She sees it and her hands can feel it. When you look at her hands closely, you can see that she is weaving a spiral of light, and if you look very closely at what her hands are weaving, you can see that it is the light from exploding nebula that come from the deepest inner depths. This is the moment and source that is the creation of images.

As she takes the dream of art and healing from the spring, she takes it to each one of us and weaves it into our hearts. There is a string inside of each strand of woven web. These strings go *from her hand and fly up as one, to each one of us, to you, up into the center of your heart. You are in the place where time and space are not limited, and these threads come up like spirals and you can see them go into infinity and they go up and down in the past, present, and the future. She holds the interlocking connections together at the side of this eternal spring. She can see us always. She sees us always. And now we can see her. She is weaving the web and holding the connections together. We can see that we are connected to many others. We are connected to everyone who is healing himself or herself with art from the beginning of time to the end of time. As we see her, we realize that we too are part of her dream. It is the ancient dream of art and healing as one. She sings to us in her eternal chant: "Each of you is an artist. Each of you is a healer."*

RECLAIMING YOUR INNER ARTIST

The guided imagery of the legend of the old woman of the springs is the first story of art and healing. In a real sense, *Creative Healing* is her song. The path to her spring is the path to creative healing. This book brings each of us to the spring where she sings, for she sings about the creativity within us. We are all artists, whether we paint, sculpt, write poetry, tell stories, dance, garden, cook, make a home, or care for someone in need. You can simply begin by journeying back to the point in which your life was the most creative. Take a few moments and close your eyes and remember these moments. Relax and you will remember your moments of creativity. You left them behind—all of us did as children. We will go back to where you were the artist. We will go back to where you left that cherished part of yourself. We will guide you to return to that moment, to reclaim yourself as an artist. You may have forgotten, so we have set up pathways of creative healing that will guide you to reunite with your most creative self. You can choose whatever medium resonates with you the most. Follow us. It is the way to spiral to your own creative source. This medium will reunite you with your artist within. It will feel natural. It will be who you are.

ART AS A WAY OF HEALING: OUR PERSONAL STORIES

We believe that at the core of the personal story told as lived experience is the truth. All through this book we tell the personal stories of patients, artists, and healers. We tell the stories of people who healed themselves with art. Within the personal story is the actual way it happened, not the theory. Like guided imagery, a personal story is something to be felt and experienced. For us, art and healing is a passion; art is a way of healing, a way of caring, and a way of knowing. How did we get here? How did we become involved in art and healing? Mary is a nurse, a wife, and a mother with three children. How did she find herself the cofounder of the Arts In Medicine program at the University of Florida? Michael is a physician, a father, a husband, and a photographer. How did he come to believe that art is a powerful healing tool for cancer patients and why did he found Art As A Healing Force? Here are their stories from the beginning. Here is how they started to become healing artists.

Mary's Story

Several years ago I was extremely ill. I was going through a very difficult divorce. I was in a rage, depressed, and extremely out of control. All the resources in my life had collapsed and I was drowning. I was not able to deal constructively with my life, with my children, or with my friends. I was in therapy, but I wasn't making any movement forward. I was surrounded by my grief and I couldn't see past it. I was in a place of darkness and despair. I remember the therapist saying to me, "It's time to do something different with your rage and your grief."

In a lucid moment, I decided to abandon my fears of being a painter, something I had always dreamed of being but had never given myself permission to be because I never felt good enough. Finally I did not put so much pressure on myself to be "good enough"; I just remembered that I had always wanted to be an artist. At that time I felt so devastated that the fear of inadequacy was minute compared to the painful loss I was experiencing. I remember the way everything happened as if it were a slow-motion movie. I walked out of the therapist's office. I was at the end of my rope. It was a drizzling-rainy kind of day. It seemed that life was going on without me. I was deeply depressed. My body was in such pain that I wanted to fall down and die. I remember walking up to a large muddy puddle. I could see my reflection in the mud. I thought about just falling down in it. I glanced up and saw a slow-moving car hesitantly driving toward me. As I looked at it, I flashed on the face of a woman I recognized. It was my friend Lee Ann. She was a painter. She came up, rolled down the car window, and said, "Why don't I take you to breakfast, and then I'll take you to my studio and you can start painting." I took out a large canvas and did not even know how to hold a brush. I looked through magazines and saw a picture of a woman who was broken and distorted. That was how I felt. I started painting. I got excited about the colors of the paint, how the shapes appeared on the paper. My painting was large and it started to look like something. Most important, it looked like my pain and it looked like how I felt. I forgot about how I felt and instead looked at how I felt. I got excited about the making of the painting. Then I got another canvas and started a series of paintings of women. They were all distorted in the beginning. I painted garish backgrounds. I took photographs of myself and I started painting myself. I became absorbed in the process and painted how I felt instead of thinking about how I felt. I began to realize I was painting my life.

Next, I created a studio space for myself and simply began painting. I painted feverishly. In the beginning, I made no attempt to define myself or my process. I painted from pure feeling states. I became absorbed in the pure expression and gesture of painting. I could completely and passionately release my energy on the canvas. The series turned out to be self-portraits. The first painting I called *Cut Out My Heart*. It was my pain, a deeply intense and dying pain. The figure was broken, distorted, diffuse, crumpled, crying, and bleeding. I painted "her." This figure had been my despair, my uncensored and purely emotional energy.

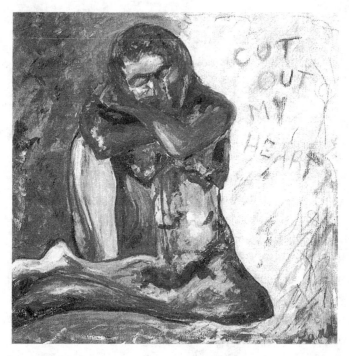

Mary Rockwood Lane, *Cut Out My Heart*. Mary Rockwood Lane healed herself of a depression by painting. She says, "The first painting I called *Cut Out My Heart*. It was my pain, a deeply intense and dying pain. The figure was broken, distorted, diffuse, crumpled, crying, and bleeding. I painted 'her.' This figure had been my despair, my uncensored and purely emotional energy. . . . As I immersed myself in painting, I not only became well, but clearly became the artist I had always wanted to be, a part of myself I had neither acknowledged nor honored. It was from this personal experience that I realized that art could be used as a vehicle for healing."

And in the moment I released this image, I stepped back and looked. Gasp. What I saw was an aspect of myself that I couldn't face, it was so ugly. Yet I felt calm and detached. I had let go on an intense emotional and physical level.

Painting is physical for me—I embody my pain as I paint it. For the first time, I was experiencing my pain in a strange and new way. As a painter, I stood in front of the canvas and was for the first time in control. I painted my emotions. I painted my body. I could feel that I was the creator of myself. I backed away, left the studio, and went home. When I returned, I saw that the image had captured and contained a moment that was now past. Then I had an incredible insight. The painting remained an object that contained an image created in genuine and immediately felt expression, and I now had moved past it. I realized that there was movement and I was witnessing my own transformation.

As I painted this series of self-portraits, in each painting I struggled with form and perspective. Metaphorically I was recreating and reconstructing my inner form and inner perspective. The external creative process mirrored my inner world. I realized that the manifestation of movement and change was powerful and that it was a process of knowing myself. As I immersed myself in painting, I not only became well, but clearly became the artist I had always wanted to be, a part of myself I had neither acknowledged nor honored. It was from this personal experience that I realized that art could be used as a vehicle for healing.

Art became a way of knowing myself through the experience of the personal pain that I painted. In seeing the painting of the pain, I could step away. I became the artist, and the series of paintings remained as the physical creation of pain. They were now my art, completely separate from me. It was a tangible experience of growing away from the place I had been when the images were painted. In essence, I became free. Then I spent time in my studio with my girlfriends painting my life. I spent two years as an artist in my studio. I painted my children playing on the beach. I painted the surrounding landscapes that I saw. I would set up still lifes on the kitchen table and I would paint the things that I loved.

Michael's Story

I was a physician on the Hopi Indian reservation that was in the center of the Navaho land. I had been sent there by the Public Health Service when my position at the National Institutes of Health was eliminated. Until then I had been a research immunogeneticist studying antibodies. Now, suddenly, I was in an emergency medicine situation that was very sad. I saw hundreds of Navaho and Hopi a day. Each patient visit could last no more than four minutes, and many of the midreservation Navaho did not speak English. Most of the patients were babies dying of dehydration from diarrhea, and we did not have a laboratory to do electrolytes. This was amazing to me. It was so dark I really could not believe it. Going to work each day I was more unhappy than I had ever been in my whole life. The way I was forced to practice medicine felt entirely wrong to me. Even when I could speak to my patients in English, as I could with the Hopi, I was excluded from their lives. All I could do was ask them how long they had been ill, what hurt, what they had been given before. All I could do was give them a prescription for medicine or refill the prescription for medicine they were taking.

The first night I was on call, two babies died of conditions that never would have killed them in the city hospital I had just come from. I felt as if we were killing the people with poor care, but each of us did the best we could under what were essentially Third World mountain conditions. Each day that I went through the motions, I became more depressed, so I left the reservation. This was very difficult for me, since had I never left anything, but I was at the end of my rope. I also realized that medicine using only drugs and surgery was not what I wanted to do, so I simply stopped doing it. I realized this had been building up for a long time, that I wanted desperately to do something in my life that allowed me to be who I was, yet after years of medical training and research, it was very hard to leave medicine and find out who I was.

So I went back to where I had done my residency. I drove up the California coast and looked for a place to live. I knew I wanted to be in the country and be on the land. I found a seaside village that called to me. Somehow it seemed like home. I walked into the real estate office and sat down and found myself telling the story of who I was. When the real estate broker heard I was a physician who was interested in the spirit, he gave me a place to live. He was a Christian Scientist and wanted a doctor around him who could treat him without using drugs when he became ill each winter. I was it. So I moved into a house overlooking the ocean and the sunset, and each day I walked on the beach and daydreamed. What would I do with my life? How could I heal the visions of the dying babies and the victims of auto accidents and the endless patients in plastic chairs moving one by one into my office, where I could only see them for four minutes? How could I heal the years of doing something I did not love and the years of abusive medical training, where I had been taught not to feel what was going on around me in people's lives?

So I daydreamed back to the last time I had been truly happy. I was a teenager; it was before medicine or even medical research had taken over my life. I was walking in the new-fallen snow at dusk. The light was soft and purple and I felt I could touch the light and move my fingers through it like thick air. It was completely still. The silence was open and I was absorbed in total peace. I was taking pictures in black and white of the stalks of grass standing upward, falling over, and looking like dancing figures in the drifts of snow. I saw the grass dancing before me in slow motion in the last light, the cold air. Space and time opened to me. That moment was the opening doorway and I went in, and in the moment of taking a picture, somehow I was free. I remembered this feeling of peace and freedom, of merging with nature and of almost disappearing into the world. This feeling was so different from the way I felt in the world of medicine I had been in for so many years. I decided, not knowing what I would do, or even who I was, that I would simply return to the last place I was truly happy.

I remembered that that was when I was a photographer, an artist. So instead of applying to another residency or going back into research, I became a photographer again and started to spend my days taking pictures of rocks on the beach. I actually defined myself as a photographer and even tried to earn my living selling photographs. I would walk each day in the dimming

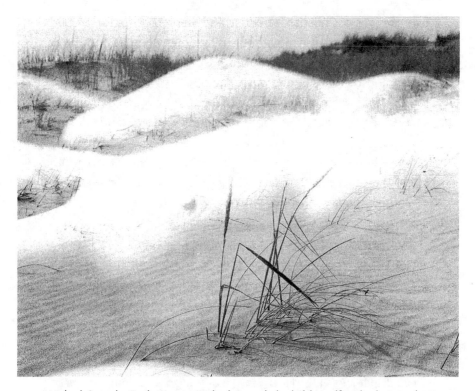

Michael Samuels, *Earth Woman.* Michael Samuels healed himself with photography. "One day I took nudes of my wife. They were very beautiful to me. Her shapes were soft and welcoming and also deeply exciting and energizing. Then I juxtaposed the negatives of the rocks with the negatives of Nancy, and my wife and the earth became one. I was deeply happy with this, and as I made my art I was slowly healed."

light and find a rock that spoke to me and take her portrait. I would look at reflections and shapes and in the looking would be enchanted. I would print the pictures and hang them and look at them deep into the night and feel the harmony of the earth.

One day I took nudes of my wife. They were very beautiful to me. Her shapes were soft and welcoming and also deeply exciting and energizing. Then I juxtaposed the negatives of the rocks with the negatives of Nancy, and my wife and the earth became one. I was deeply happy with this, and as I made my art I was slowly healed of medical school and the pain I saw there. I was healed of all my memories of people's sadness and abuse, and the dying babies. I was healed from the emptiness of the way doctors treated patients and how impersonal the work was in hospitals and how dark the world of being sick and only being looked at as a body was. I started to think about creating my life anew, making my life as art.

Nancy and I built our home together, and to finance this I started working as a physician again. But this time I was different. I used meditation techniques I had learned, I spent time with my patients, listening to their stories, and I started to do relaxation and guided imagery as part of allopathic medicine. I had changed. My medicine had changed. My way of seeing and my way of being had changed. Looking back on this story, it seems to me that my artist within came and got me in my darkest moment and healed me. And when it happened, it just happened. I did not heal myself; I was healed by my photography.

Years later, as my wife was having a bone marrow transplant for breast cancer, I wrote a journal about the experience, and that probably saved my life then. I was staying in her hospital room for the five weeks the procedure took. Watching her undergo this difficult procedure and worrying about its complications was as hard as anything I had ever done. And again my inner artist emerged. For reasons I didn't know, I decided to bring a laptop into her room and write each day. And each day I awakened to the world of my story and the world of her transplant. What I found was that each day I would see what was happening to her and me, and I would see it out of the eyes of myself as the writer artist. I would also see her spirit, and somehow each day I would give thanks for seeing it. Instead of being sad or being a crisis report, my journal became deeply spiritual. It became a story of bravery and of Nancy as my teacher. The artist within had changed my eyes. Each time I wrote, I could see her differently and see what was happening to us in a way that was sustaining for me and not depressing. Somehow my vision was of her beauty, not of her suffering, and that is the vision I hold even to this day.

HOW DOES THE ART OF HEALING RELATE TO HEALING ART?

Creative healing brings forth an illuminated aspect of ourselves in everything that we do. This book is an activity. It is about becoming illuminated and coming out of concealment. For people who want to be healed, there is a moment in their lives where they can see themselves anew. There is a moment when you drive along the road and see the sun-dappled leaves, their green richness, and see yourself in it. Creative healing brings on a shift in experience. For each person there is the vision that stands out in his or her life. It can be a memory of a spiritual vision, a time with our families, or the making of art. In this book, we will take you to that vision and slow it down so you can see it more clearly. That is what art does. We will look more closely and more slowly, in between the moments, in between our breaths.

Creative healing is about returning to the source of healing, and regeneration. It is programmed from the spirit to the mind to the body. This book will help you tap into the creative source of healing in a spiritual way. This book will be like a seed that has given birth. You have this deep capacity for transformation. You spiral inward to make contact with your healing energy. Any intentional act to heal yourself will access it. We will use the force of your passionate creativity, and in this manner we will intentionally use art to manifest forms that express healing. We will use art to express light, anger, joy, and change. We will use art to express yourself.

A GUIDED IMAGERY EXERCISE TO CONTACT YOUR INNER HEALER

This next guided imagery takes you deep inside yourself to the place where images come from, to the place where you make art, and to the place where you heal. This imagery is different from the imagery of the old woman of the springs. It does not tell a story. It takes you into a visual place of being inside your body. It takes you into your own healing physiology. It takes you into the meditative space where time and space are changed and where art and healing are one.

Close your eyes; let your breathing get slower and deeper; relax. All you have to do now is let yourself go into your imagination, into your mind's eye. Let yourself read these words and just be with them and everything will happen by itself. There is nothing to do. Your mind will take you where you need to be with your imagination. All you need to do is rest.

Let's picture in our mind's eye going inward on a journey on a sacred spiral. The spiral is very ancient. It comes from ancient memories of our birth and our rebirth. The spiral is how we emerged in the birth canal. As we were born, we all turned and rotated and went downward toward the light. As we die, we all spiral and turn and go upward toward the light. It is all the same, all deep within our remembrances, deep within our souls. In mythology, the spiral is the movement of going into the center of all energy. In nature, spirals are the basic forms of space and time; they are in stars, in light, in nebula and galaxies, in seashells.

Now see and feel your body as made of energy and movement. Inside it you can see colors and flow; you can see channels and fluids moving. Now look inside your body and see the spirals of motion that are within you. There are small ones in the cells, larger ones in the organs, and a larger one within your whole body. They do not necessarily correspond to anatomical body parts; they are just the beauty within us. See and feel the spirals within your body merging with each other. See and feel your spirals and those of your loved ones. See how your spirals touch your children, your loved ones. See and feel the spirals merge when you make love. The vortexes within all of us are constantly in movement, constantly interacting with the environment and one another. We are all born on the sacred spiral. and we spiral forever in time and space, like the planet earth spirals around the sun. We spiral in orbits of space and time. The universal movement is within us and outside us; it is contracting and expanding, breathing in and breathing out. The spiral goes beyond ordinary time and space, and within the spiral you can connect to ancient healing spirits that will be your helpers and your guides. As you spiral inward to a deeper place inside of yourself, you will pass through a membrane to the center of your own heart and you will feel the pulsating of the universe from the very center of yourself and you will realize that you are interconnected with everything.

In the center of your heart is the source of love, of passion and desire. There are no forms there, and all forms emerge from it. It is the way the ancient ones knew the earth. It is the place that is shared with all others, where there is no thought or emotions. It is the place that is sacred. It is the source of your life and the place where you are one with your creator. This is the place within you that is the source from which everything emerges. You are now inside the membrane.

The membrane holds the space between the inner and outer world; it always separates the space of the two sides. The membrane is a metaphor for going from the outer world to the inner world. It is chosen as the metaphor because in the outer world, the membrane always separates two sides. In our bodies, the membrane is the sac around the amniotic fluid before birth. All cells have it; all birth is through it. It is like a veil. At any given moment on the membrane it emerges; the source of life comes from the other side of the membrane. Outside is the outer world of your body, your family, your environment, all the things that you know. You are now across the membrane, inside your heart in the inner world, which is spirit, formless, your source, your source of creativity. In the membrane is something between the inner and outer worlds. You can always access the place inside you through your art. In the act of your passion and your creativity, you can spiral to this place that is your inner source. You can always return to this place through the tangible world. This moment or place resonates and spirals throughout your experience of who you are and goes through all the experiences in your life. You are inside the membrane in a place where you are totally free. When you return from this imagery you will go to your living experience, to the place of tangibles. This is the point from which you will start to get well. Your illness may be the place where you feel that all your resources may have ended and all is gone. It is the place to return to your desire to live, to be fully alive, and to be happy. The point is to get well. This is the choice—to heal yourself. The artist is a way of healing.

Now rest a moment and let yourself become aware of your breathing. Notice that there is a moment between breaths. There is a pause, a moment of suspended animation. There is a moment where you are not actually breathing; you just are. Move into this space with the intention to heal. Say to yourself, "I am starting from this place with the intention to do what I have always wanted to do in my life." This is a prayer. In this moment you shift into being one with your creator, one with your source, and then you begin to breathe in and out. You breathe in and out to move into any other dimension. The process is the pathway. Now you are on the pathway. Art is the way. All that was the unconscious is now conscious, and you can see deeply that there is a wisdom and a truth to what you are doing in your creation. You can see the glimpse of it in your heart. You heal instantly by the glimpse of what is the miracle of your life, and what you are in this moment emerges as the purest and most beautiful of forms. You are now the artist. You are beautiful and passionate. You are creative. What is now important is having faith in your own creativity. You have become one with your artist. This artist is the pathway to the healer.

In this guided imagery exercise, you have become an artist. From now on, your artist is on the pathway to your healer, the healer within. This artist will activate the pathway of continuous creation. Your objective as an artist is to make forms. You make art in forms that are fluid. You do not need to understand these forms; you only need to flow with them. Flow with your own spiral of creativity. Inherent is constant change, constant beauty, the ability to love. You see this. Inherent in the creative is the ability to be formed.

Instead of illness teaching you about limits, your artist can take you into freedom and passionate creativity. You are powerful. You are now the creator. You go into the opposite of illness, you go into freedom, creativity, limitlessness. Then you become empowered. As the artist, you stand in front of yourself. You can see who you are. You have changed as an artist. You will not stay the same; you will grow and change. Now you realize that art is the way to open the door again and again to something new and different. You realize that you harness the creative energy inside you and therefore can influence what happens to you in your life. This energy can deeply affect your personal inner world, if not necessarily the outer one. It is exhilarating to feel creativity, to experience the empowerment that comes from the ability to create. That is the source of the life change.

Next you realize that the only way to keep the flow going is to let art come through you into the outer world. Let it go out, let it flow. It comes from love. It is about cultivation and grace. You offer yourself to be connected to thoughts. You offer yourself to others. You allow yourself to love yourself and be seen and give someone the wonderful opportunity to love you back. It is not an outcome; it is a continuous process. We give from the center of our hearts to the center of another's. The first path is to heal yourself; the next path is to heal others. By knowing this path, you share it with others. Know that we are on the path of the healer. This path is not dependent on traditions. It is just from the center of your own heart. Listen. Honor the creative expression. With acceptance, honor the fullest expression of yourself. Know that constant transformation and healing are deeper than our body; they are in the center of our heart and soul.

| THREE |

STORY TIME: THE HISTORY OF ART AND HEALING

The story of art and healing is an ancient one. It tells of how people have used art to heal themselves from the time of the hunter-gatherer human culture to the time of the newest programs in hospitals today. This story grounds you in the flow of your past, present, and future; it connects you to your ancestors. It shows you that you are a part of a great tradition that has gone on since the beginning of both art and healing. We include this chapter on the story of art and healing to give you increased faith in using art to heal by knowing that this new field is actually the oldest healing there is. What is the main thing we can learn from listening to the stories of the first artist healers? That healing with art is as old as being a mother and that the first artist and the first healer were one person and they were just like you; they had your body, your mind, and your spirit. This powerful tool for healing has been used forever. Now you can use it, too.

THE STORY OF ART AND HEALING

What is the story of art and healing? To summarize, it is a journey from the nurturing care of a mother singing a lullaby to a hunter in a cave preparing

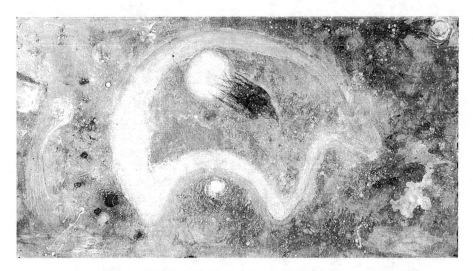

Erica Swadley, *Fire on Her Moon*. Healing artists are a part of the great tradition of the shaman/artist/healer that has gone on since the beginning of both art and healing. Erica says, "A great she-bear seemed to be hanging around me, breathing over my right shoulder, expecting something from me. I felt her hot breath dampening my hair and neck. A small image of her, cast in the sky with the moon and a raven in her belly, imprinted itself and wouldn't let go until I had painted it and repainted it."

his vision of the hunt. It moves from the woman mystic doing a ritual around childbirth to the tribal peoples who danced together to heal. It journeys from the shaman as a healer specialist of the inner world to the sacred artist and healer of Buddhism, Judaism, Christianity, and all other religions. It reaches the modern artist whose paintings show us another view of changing space and time and finally ends up in the present day, where artists and healers use art to heal themselves, others, and the earth. The journey sounds long, and there are large jumps between the stages as we describe them. The separations, however, are artificial. The evolution happened in a more complicated and nuanced way, but the major points add up the same. One person makes art and goes inward and frees the inner healer. The process is ordinary and visionary at once. We are still every one of the heroes in these stories. We are parents, spiritual people, and modern-day artist healers. As we make healing art, we add our stories to the ongoing saga. We are the healing artists. As we make art, we remember who we are.

IN THE BEGINNING WAS THE MOTHER

At the beginning of art and healing is the simple story of a mother. As she sat holding her baby in her arms, she sang a lullaby. We believe that the first piece of healing art was the lullaby of a mother to her baby. And that probably started before the baby was even born. Within the uterus, the unborn baby could hear his mother singing, he could see soft colors; she could feel her mother dancing and making love. Art as healing came from mothering and loving. After the baby was born, as the mother took care of her baby, she still sang songs. She decorated the baby's cradle board, she made her beautiful clothing, she rocked him to sleep in a carved cradle.

When the baby was ill, which was common in ancient times, the mother's songs became more serious; they turned into chants and prayers. We can imagine that after hours of singing, she would see spirits and hear songs from the wind or from the night. She would sing these new songs to her baby. Anthropology tells us that in ancient times women believed that there were spirits, helpers, forces, or powers who could help heal a baby, so mothers sang and chanted to bring these spirits to their lovingly carved cradles. The fathers, too, naturally used art to heal. When the baby was ill, he told stories and made believe he was a great bear. Ancient stories tell us that fathers even believed that they could contact a bear spirit to help their babies heal. The mother might say a prayer and carve a doll who was a protector or an ancestor. African mothers to this day carve amulets to protect their babies and to honor ancestors and babies they have lost. So healing with art was always about love and spirituality. Each of us can still be healers in this way now.

We believe that the first healing art was as natural as mothering; it came from the deep love of a mother for her baby. This could be why most healing artists today are women and why most healing traditions using art throughout history have involved mystical women. Woman mystics are pioneers, delving deep into the mysteries of the inner world. You can imagine a distant time when women would get together in a circle and sing to one of their own who was grieving from a loss or dance with a woman who was about to give birth. The traditions of childbirth were rich with art: women midwives sang, instructed mothers to dance, and made amulets to protect mothers-to-be from dangers that in ancient times were very real. Adorning their bodies, painting, tattooing, and scarification were all part of ancient healing practices and of a woman's everyday life. Art was a way of caring.

The first art made of a woman is believed to have been the Venus of Magellen. This magnificent sculpture portrays a woman in her most beautiful shape. Her breasts are large and pendulous, her belly huge and round. In the art she looks like she has given birth to the earth and is breastfeeding it daily. This sculpture embodies fertility, fecundity, and the power to create life. Imagine a man or a woman making this sculpture during a ceremonial ritual. Such images were believed to be ritual objects for fertility and childbirth, or simply to represent the reverence for the life force itself, which was seen as Her. Amulets of these figures were carried to protect a person or help a woman create babies, to enhance her fertility, and to heal the earth.

The first mothers made their healing art in private with their babies. As a woman sat singing to her sick baby, she might make up a story that would explain what illness was about or what had caused the problem. This story would be the subject of the healing art, of the song, of the amulet. This art was not often made of materials that lasted and is probably lost to recorded history. Later, groups of women told these stories over and over again, and they became the culture's theories of illness and the subject of rituals performed in healing groups. Men, too, would tell stories, dance, sing, and build theories of illness that became the basis of healing rituals or ceremonies.

As the rituals grew and became more elaborate, they probably resembled today's theatrical performances. They were a mixture of elaborate costumes, stories, songs, and drama. People believed that this ritual would bring in the healing spirits and heal their loved ones. In ancient times and even now, all cultures except ours have believed that illness is caused by being out of harmony with spiritual forces. For that reason, the art used in healing tended to be spiritual in nature. It often portrayed spirits or protectors or even ancestors who had died and thus lived in the world of the spirits. Other healing art was about a person's life, about a hunt or a journey or a place they loved. But one thing is clear from these stories—the art was transformational. It was done to accomplish something, to heal, to soothe, to love. It was done to make the hunt successful, to make the land fertile, to control the weather, and to heal. Yes, art was decoration, but its main function was transformative: to create balance and to heal.

THE CAVE MAN AND WOMAN AND THE ANIMALS

Most art historians consider cave paintings to be the earliest form of recorded art. On the walls of the cave in Tres Friers in southern France, magnificent paintings portray a human with large circled eyes wearing a headdress with tall antlers, possibly representing a hunter or a shaman. These paintings are thought to portray magical visions to improve the hunt. This would make sense, for the early hunter knew his animals deeply. To be able to hunt animals with a spear, he had to get close, close enough to literally touch their bodies. To do that, he had to know their habits, trails, ways of moving, what they ate, where they found water. He could almost see out of the animal's eyes, and when he killed the animal he worshiped it as if it had offered him its body. The hunter honored the animal's spirit and became one with it. He knew the animal like he knew himself. When the animal died, its spirit was often believed to enter into the hunter, and then he would know the animal even better. He would become an even more powerful hunter.

You can imagine the early cave man or woman dancing in a dark cave lit only by fire. You can picture him or her painting pictures of the dancers in their wild headdresses on the walls. It is theorized that the hunter believed that when he dressed as the animal he became the animal. He could speak to the spirit and ask it to come to him in the hunt. It was a spiritual union of human and animal that spoke of reverence and interdependence. After all, we share the same DNA with the animals. We have hearts like they do, breathe like they do; they are our brothers and sisters. The experience of "becoming" the animal was primary to the making of this ancient art. Hunters would paint themselves with animal blood and dung and transform themselves into the very creatures they hunted. Through their art, they became more powerful and better able to hunt and feed their people.

DANCING TO FREE OUR BOILING ENERGY

One of the most beautiful stories of art and healing comes from the Kalihari Bushman people of the African desert. The Bushmen are a people living today as hunter-gatherers. Looking at them may yield exciting clues about how people used art and healing for thousands of years. For 99 percent of human evolution, humans were hunter-gatherer peoples. Richard Katz of the Harvard University Kalihari project visited these people and wrote about their healing rituals in his book *Boiling Energy*. He describes how the Bushmen would dance all night several nights a week. They believed that dance freed up the boiling energy within them and was the way to heal. During the dance ritual, their bodies became incredibly hot and enormous energy came up from within them. These techniques often caused their illness to subside. Sometimes they would go into a trance after dancing for hours, and people around them would touch them and help them. This community healing ritual was an ordinary part of Bushman life, not something special or artificial. It fit in with the people's worldview and probably evolved over thousands of years.

The healing dancing of the Bushmen has several important characteristics in the story of art and healing. First, the dance—the art—was done by everyone. There was no figure who did something to you. There were people who led the dance, but the healing was done by the dancing itself. The physical movements freed the healing energy. So in a very real sense, the dancers became their own healing artists. Each person made the art that freed his or her inner healer. Second, people did not separate out "art" and "healing." Their healing dancing was simply a freeing of energy, a transformation. It was not just for entertainment, although it certainly was the most exciting thing they could do. Dance and healing were one. We cannot say the dance caused healing—it simply was healing.

A GUIDED IMAGERY FOR FREEING BOILING ENERGY

This imagery lets you picture in your imagination what it must have been like to be among the hunter-gatherers who healed themselves with dance.

Close your eyes; relax; let your breathing slow down; take several deep breaths; let your abdomen rise and fall. Now imagine that you are on a plain, a rolling prairie. Look up and you can see more stars than you have ever seen before. The whole sky is like an inverted bowl; the stars are like other worlds. The air feels soft on your skin. Your breathing feels deep. You touch your feet to the ground and feel the soft earth. You know that this is a special vision, and you feel deeply as if you have been in this sacred place many times before.

Let yourself be on the great plain under the stars on a beautiful clear night. The mountains shine in the distance, and the grazing animals cover the plains like distant trees. All your friends and relatives are around you; in fact, all the people you know and have ever known are there. You are there to dance—you do this several times a week. People around you start to dance, to move, to shake. Music starts, and drums beat all around you. You know you are here to heal, to free your boiling energy. Suddenly you can feel yourself dancing, spinning and whirling with all your people. You feel your body getting hot and you feel the energy rising within you. You feel yourself going round and round in larger and smaller circles, and as you spin you feel yourself go deep into the spinning and deep into yourself. Soon the stars and the plains and the animals are forgotten and you see yourself as if you are above you. You are just beautiful, and as you see yourself dancing you can see red lines of energy shooting up from the base of your spine and moving all throughout your body. You dance for hours and you feel looser and looser and more and more wonderful and in the crystal dawn you are free and relaxed. You feel as if you are in perfect balance with the whole world and with all your people.

Then you see a person you know as a lead dancer. That person comes up to you and you fall into his or her arms. And as you fall the dancer holds you and pushes on your body where it had hurt. The healing energy gets even brighter and more beautiful. You are healed, whole, alive, and full. You go back to your house and you see it is a part of the prairie. You lie down to sleep and you vibrate like the mountains, you move like the winds, you shine like the stars themselves. And you remember that you do this almost every night; it is the way you keep well and heal. It is an important part of your life. Now come back into your own room and awaken to your usual state of mind. You can see your bedroom or couch and you can see the furniture and the things that usually surround you. You can bring this vision back with you and you can dance to heal whenever you want to. You have this memory deep within your cells. You can be your own artist healer. You can bring back these feelings of freeing your inner energy and use them when-ever you want to, in imagery space or as a dancer. This is how healing with art feels; this is how it always felt.

THE FIRST ARTIST AND THE FIRST HEALER WERE ONE PERSON: THE SHAMAN

The next stage in the story of art and healing comes from the birth of shamanism. Shamanism is a cultural practice where a person goes into another world (which psychologists now see as that person's inner world or imagina-tion) and sees spirits, gods, or forces. The spirits are communicated with and wield influence to heal, to let a person free, to let animals come to a hunt, to control the wind or sea, to influence fertility, to change the world. It is our belief that the shaman evolved from the ordinary person making art. When you make art you concentrate deeply; you go into a creative place inside you and have ideas or visions or thoughts. From these inner meditations, you create a work of art. Remember the story of the mother who sees spirits after hours of singing to her sick baby? That is all shamanism is. The creative trance takes you to the inner world, where you are different.

In the Bushman culture every person in the tribe danced and went into a trance and felt the boiling energy come from within them. Over time, however, the ancient tribal culture changed. As the hunter-gatherer cultures became more complicated, people tended to specialize. Everyone did not dance three times a week, because they were out hunting or building houses or gathering food for a larger group. And as the people stopped making art several times a week, they lost their ability to see into their own inner world. They simply got out of practice. Something else took their attention. But there were still individuals who danced and made amulets and sang and went into trances and saw spirits in the inner world. Since the main cause of illness in all the cultures in the world was believed to be spiritual, these individuals were valued and became experts in the act of seeing within. Mercea Eliade, the eminent University of Chicago history of religions scholar, said that a shaman was a specialist in seeing spirits, the first specialist in the soul. Similarly, in contemporary times, the healing artist is a medical specialist in restoring the body and soul.

Shamans received their calling by having a dream or vision, by inheriting the position from a relative, or by healing themselves from an illness. Generally, the ability to see visions or to dream was the major requirement. Human culture had gone from a place where everyone was an artist healer to a place where some people who were naturally gifted at it did it for the group. But two of the main characteristics of early art and healing still remained. First, art and healing were still one; they just were not being done by everyone. The shaman was thus the first artist and the first healer. And second, in the time of the shaman, art was still transformational. Art was made to heal or to hunt. In that sense, all of us who are healing ourselves with art are modern shamans.

Eventually in tribal cultures, music and dance were combined with costumes and storytelling and with objects and paintings in the creation of a ritual we would now call theater or performance art. In ancient times, this ritual was sacred and it was part of the culture's healing practices. In ancient cultures, it was believed that illness was caused by spirits or forces and that the only way to contact the spirits was by a shaman going into a trance. In the trance, the shaman saw the spirits, talked them into releasing the illness or the person, and came back to the tribe and told the story of the journey. Ancient shamans did not venture inward without their powerful animal

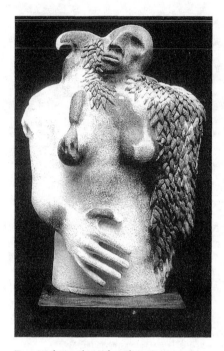

Tom Wolver, *She Who Flies*. Contemporary artists make images of animal transformations that are as compelling as those made thousands of years ago. Tom says, "The shapes that I call up dwell in a deep, primal region that I have been granted access to into the shadow world. As an artist, it is my responsibility to willingly descend, to shine a light in those dark places, to make a record of those images, and, finally, to bring these images back to the surface of consciousness intact. My vision is a mythical one, on the journey through the 'dark' side to eventual healing."

spirits to guide them. Much art was made by the shamans portraying their journeys, and thus art often contained images of animals, spirits, canoes, shamans, skeletons, plants, gods, and goddesses. All these images were actually seen by the shaman in the inner world and were painted, sculpted, and danced as they were seen. In a very real sense, shamanic art was realistic. It portrayed real experiences that the shaman had and did so as a means of communication. The art was also believed to have power in itself: the images were believed to contain part of the power of the object portrayed.

Art and healing were one in the time of the shaman. Why was this so? There was no art as such, no art as an activity separate from communicating with the spirits and accessing their power. The first healing art of the shaman was about embodiment, about becoming the spirit or animal, about being it as totally as the shaman could. The second way art and healing were one was based on sharing. When healers wanted to share their experience with the patient or the village, they told the story. The way they made the story come vividly alive for people, it became a kind of early theater.

Much later, native peoples would carve stone sculptures of human-animal transformations. Often the pieces would portray a shaman with a bear head or a woman with owl wings or even a dancing shaman with bear claws and an owl's face. Native peoples say that the transformation pieces illustrate the stories shamans told of turning into animals, seeing out of an animal's eyes, taking on the animal spirit. The carvings enabled the people to share the experience and see what the shaman had seen. The pieces would often be carried by shamans in their pockets or hung on their costumes. It was believed that the pieces gave the shaman power by holding the energy of the spirit animal transformation.

As human culture changed, specialization became more and more extreme. Later, in agricultural societies, certain people made art and certain people concentrated on healing. Art and healing became separated more and more, and each discipline became more specialized. The person who did each action became a different person who was then called an "artist" or a "healer." But there were always those of us who held onto the original vision of art and healing as one. Some artists painted or sculpted their sacred visions, and these visions were seen as deeply healing. But the main cultural trend was clear: art and healing were becoming two different actions. They were done by two different people. Further specialization had arrived.

Today, artist healers still heal by art from visions of healing forces. When you dance, you can still free the healing energy. When you paint, you can still paint healing forces. When you write, you can still tell your own story of how you are healing.

THE OLD WOMAN OF THE SPRINGS: HOW ART AND HEALING WERE BORN

As we told you earlier, the old woman of the springs was the mother of all forms on earth. As we tell more and more of her story, she tells us more about how art and healing were born. In this chapter of her story, she tells us how she gave birth to the first art, poetry, music, and dance and to the first artist healer.

> Now go back in your mind to the story of the old woman of the springs. Go back to the forest, the path, the circular turquoise spring. And as she weaves the earth from her dreams, she sings to us. Close your eyes and listen to her song: "Listen to my song my children. I will tell you the story of how art and healing were born. It is the oldest story. It is a story tied to the story of who

you are and where you came from. It is a story about your origins. It is a creation story. Listen, listen to my tale.

"From deep within my most ancient memories, from far within my deepest love, my dream emerges. Oh, I put my hands deep inside my own body, into the stars, into the night, into the seas, into the forests, and I pull out the strands of the dream, I pull out the animals of the four directions, I pull out their spirits, I pull out time and space, I pull out my peoples." And as you listened to her, she reached into herself, she who was all there was, except for the spring, and she pulled out time and space and she pulled out the four directions and she pulled out the animals' spirits and she pulled out the first peoples.

And the first peoples rested and slept and they stirred and stretched and they stood up on their legs and they looked around. They saw the spring and they saw her weaving them still and they were amazed and joyful and they opened their mouths and a song came out and they moved and it was dance and they touched their fingers to the earth and it was their visions and they spoke and it was the first poem. And the first peoples made art with their first breaths and they saw her always above them, dreaming them, and they were at peace.

She loved them perfectly, of course, and she put this memory deep within them and knew that they would need this connection later when they became afraid. And then the old woman saw them grow and prosper and she saw them start to make objects and hunt and farm, and she saw them stop making art and stop seeing her. And she sat one day and went deep into her heart and pulled out a special silver thread, and it was the thread of her own memory and it was the thread of art and healing as one and it was the thread that led to her heart, too. She pulled out this thread and she put it into each of the first people's *hearts and it connected them to her because she could see that they were going away. And she cried and she knew it was time and she knew, too, that they would be coming home, for that is the way the story went in each of the cycles of the world.*

And there was born to these peoples those who always saw the silver threads and always heard her song and always saw her face. They were the dreamers and they were inside and outside at once and they were also the first artist and the first healer. Because they were on her threads, they were the first artist and the first healer as one person. They were the first shaman, the first shamaness, the first seer of visions, the first specialist in the soul. For as the peoples became busy they saw outward more, inward less, and finally could only see outward by themselves and needed help to see inward, and the help was the shaman and the shamaness.

THE POWER OF THE SPRINGS

This ancient story of the old woman and the springs is true. It is paralleled in anthropology, in art history, and in the history of religions. And it is paralleled in our own body's physiology and in our memories of hearing sounds and seeing colors in utero and of birth. Every culture has a healing spring and a woman who watches over it. Native cultures tell us that the woman of the springs sits above each spring and speaks of the secrets of the earth. They tell us that all the springs are connected and the same woman speaks to everyone at each spring. They tell us that there are women in the tribe who still can understand the voice of the old woman of the springs. They say that if you listen, her voice can be heard next to any spring. Lourdes in France and Tinos in Greece are two of thousands of springs that are places of healing pilgrimages today. There are many springs that the Virgin Mary has shown to people in visions.

Stone circles and megaliths also have always been associated with healing rituals. Ley lines cross the earth with the energies of healing and in England are believed to be male and female, and where they cross they join.

Sacred spots on earth have always been associated with healing energy and have been worshiped in ancient times, tribal times, and recent times. In one spot, often next to a spring, there will be an Indian mound, a church, and a new-age pilgrimage site. She still speaks to us, though, the ancient woman of the springs ... she does.

EGYPTIAN AND SUMERIAN ART

When agricultural societies became large and specialized, the art still was transformational. In the art of the first agricultural peoples, one of the main sources of imagery was the gods and goddesses. Healing gods were portrayed in human and animal forms. The images were made to show the people what the gods looked like, so they could see them themselves and receive power themselves. The huge statues of gods and goddesses were believed to influence the harvest, the weather, fertility, and healing. The making of these sculptures was from visions seen by priests and was deeply sacred. The kings were buried with these works of art, which were believed to influence the afterlife. The Sumerian and Egyptian cultures had a deep belief in mental imagery influencing outer reality. Hermetic philosophy believed that a mental image became real in the outer world if accompanied by prayers and that the art helped make the prayers more alive and real. The visions of the gods in their animal forms were believed to reveal deeper incarnations of the gods that were extremely powerful.

SACRED ART AND SACRED HEALING

As shamanism spread and became incorporated into mainstream religion, healing art also became part of religious art. As Judaism developed, it held the belief that idols were not to be made of God. Faith was to be the way of worship, and imagery that portrayed the deity was considered profane. But there was much sacred art in Judaism. Torahs, temples, and shawls have the design of the star of David and also portraits of Abraham and Moses and historical events from the Bible. Again these images helped share the visions of the prophets with the people, but they were not believed to have primary power by the Jewish people. In Judaism, they were believed to represent the power of God in art forms.

Christian and Buddhist art were based on the principle that meditating on images or listening to certain sounds could put a person in a sacred state that would be healing. Now art and healing were two: the artist was a specialist in making art and the healer in healing. But because scientific healing had not yet been born, both art and healing remained spiritual. The next movement in art was largely spiritual. Imagery in both Christian and Buddhist art depicted sacred stories drawn or sculpted from the visions of artist mystics. The healers still believed in a spiritual cause of illness, but the model of the one figure, the shaman healer, was replaced in large agricultural cultures by the separate roles of the sacred artist and the sacred healer. Today, people who are ill use art from their religion to heal. Patients in hospital rooms put up crosses, icons, stars of David, and Buddhas and pray to them to heal. Spiritual healing art is used extensively around the world as a primary healing tool, as it has been for centuries.

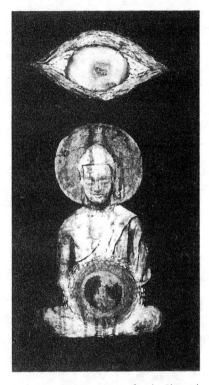

Beth Ames Swartz, *A Story for the Eleventh Hour*. The healing artist is the sacred image maker of contemporary times. Beth Ames says, "I am committed to creating work that can make a difference in our lives, that is intentionally healing in its imagery and contributes to an environment of renewal. I help to heal myself by doing art! The Buddha and the all-seeing eye are icons symbolizing our race's potential for compassion and enlightened behavior."

TIBETAN BUDDHIST ART

Tibetan Buddhist art gives us the most elaborate description of how art heals. People who heal themselves with art use a process similar to that of a Buddhist artist who makes art. They make an image that is believed to have power and share a vision of healing. The doctrines of Buddhism are the most detailed and intricate, and the art itself the most technical. For Buddhism, art is a spiritual "high technology" of healing that takes place in a sacred spiritual geography. Art in Tibetan Buddhism is sacred and healing. In Buddhism, it is believed that a person's life itself can be an art that can communicate the vision of enlightenment and inspire others to find relief and happiness. In this view, for a fully enlightened being the only goal for any type of art is liberating others—healing others from suffering.

The seeds of art as healing are contained in the central doctrine of Buddhism itself. According to this doctrine, when one becomes a Buddha, one is transformed into three bodies. The first is the Truth Body, which is the experience of wisdom. The second is the Beatific Body, which is the experience of bliss. The third is the Emanation Body, which is the way bliss and wisdom are communicated to others. The Emanation Body is divided into three bodies. The first is the Supreme Emanation Body of the Buddha's to help others. The second is the Incarnational Emanation Body of teachers to help others. The third is the Artistic Emanation Body, made up of anything that represents enlightenment. This is the aspect that particularly applies to us here. The Artistic Emanation Body is made up of all the sacred art and the artists who create it. Literature, visual arts, and sculpture that represent the sacred life of the Buddha are all crucial in helping people attain liberation. It is believed that Buddha could not even begin his task of liberating people until their imaginations were opened up to the possibility of enlightenment by looking at art. So art is crucial to the whole structure of Buddhism. It is nothing less than the way individuals can see, hear, listen, understand, and know how a new reality of enlightenment is possible for them in their life. Art is the way wisdom and bliss are communicated to others.

In Buddhism, healing is seen as total well-being and expanded creativity of enlightenment. It is much more than the absence of disease. So for Buddhism, art is the creative energy that manifests in order to heal; it is the precious window into enlightenment, into the other world. In this way, art is viewed as a gift of the enlightened ones, of the gods. It is also believed that art makes itself when done perfectly: the gods produce "wisdom duplicates" of themselves that merge with the sculpture. Thus, Tibetans believe that a sculpture transmits a living presence and that its power can be increased by prayer and ritual.

For the Tibetans, the most important healing art is the life you live. Your Artistic Emanation Body is the most powerful art form, the most powerful artistic emanation. For your life to be healing art, you must live with the intent to heal in every breath. The second most important art is literature. Songs, epics, poems, tales, and legends are believed to be a direct path to your imagination, a way to let you picture enlightenment directly. Next in importance is music. Tibetans believe that harmony and vibration affect your heart directly. Chants are believed to open the heart, to heal and inspire. Architecture is also important. It can create sacred geography, sacred space. It designs mandalas, which convey delight, security, and exaltation. Deities are seen at precise places within the architecture, the sacred building serving as their home. Of course, the most elaborate structures that can ever be built are those we create in our minds with guided imagery. They are incredibly intricate and exact representations of heavenly abodes.

Sculpture is a way to embody yourself as a god. As you picture the icon, you energize the mental image until you are merged with it and become it. The Tibetan Buddhist first pictures the deity in his or her mind and then in the icon. The mind form is the most powerful. Buddhists visualize themselves being made anew—being born, as it were—as the deity. It takes the utmost discipline and practice to manifest as an enlightened being. Paintings also are seen as windows into the enlightened world. They are exact representations of the Buddha world and must be painted perfectly to be of optimal use.

In Tibetan Buddhism, art is a direct flowing out from the enlightened spaces of Buddha. It gives a person a way to be embodied as an enlightened one, and that is how healing occurs. As you are enlightened, you are healed. This does not always involve curing, since everyone dies, including Buddha and the Dalai Lama. Death in Buddhism is a doorway to enlightenment and the gateway to the next reincarnation, so it is not in itself frightening or a thing to be avoided. This view is directly applicable to our own experience—even among those of us who are not Buddhists. We can look at sacred art and picture the images in our mind's eye and help heal ourselves, too. Or we can hold any image that we believe will heal us and meditate on it. This is the Buddhist tradition of healing art. As healing artists, we each follow the Buddhist practice of helping others achieve well-being.

Art has always been a way of enhancing our ordinary lives. Art has been integral to religion and society. From the stone circles in ancient times to churches in more recent times, art grounded the cultures in the spiritual world. Art was also the ordinariness of making bowls, baskets, and household objects that expressed the beautiful forms of life. Art has always been the way people have contemplated their reverence and awe for life and human spirit. As artists and as healers, we have discovered in our own lives, and in the lives of our patients, that art and healing are one. The original marriage of the two disciplines is still alive, and the power of the union is able to heal us as it did in the crystal dawn when our ancestors danced as early humans.

So art has gone from a mother's care and lullaby to advanced therapeutics. It has gone from love and spirituality in caring to love and spirituality in healing. It is the oldest healing and art, and the newest body-mind-spirit healing technique. We have come full circle, full spiral. But the essential component that remains in art and healing is the reconnection of art and science. Art and science split when knowledge development was necessary for modern medicine to be born. Then science became focused on linear logic and separated from spiritual practice. Art, spirituality, and science split. This allowed for growth of science and the concepts of understanding the body and its physiology. Art became more connected to spirit and lost its place in healing. Now is the time for art and healing to reunite as one. You are the healing artist today as your ancestors were in the beginning of each of our stories.

FOUR

How Art Heals: The Physiology of Art and Healing

The spirit, mind, and body are one, and an image of art that comes from the spirit and is seen in the mind affects the body. In that view, we are made to heal ourselves with art. Our bodies have evolved to do this. This is our evolutionary neurobiology; it is that simple. When we experience art, our body's self-healing mechanisms are released to work at their best. So if you are a woman with breast cancer who wants to heal herself with art, it's important to understand that the process of making art profoundly changes your spiritual state and your mental state and thereby helps your immune system to get rid of the cancer cells. When people have cancer, their body's white blood cells eat the cancer cells. Otherwise, no one would heal. Chemotherapy kills many cells, but your body kills the rest. When you make art, your immune system is freed; its function is enhanced. Your attitude is changed, your quality of life improved, and, we believe, your chance of curing the cancer improved. Come with us and listen to the stories about the physiology of art and healing.

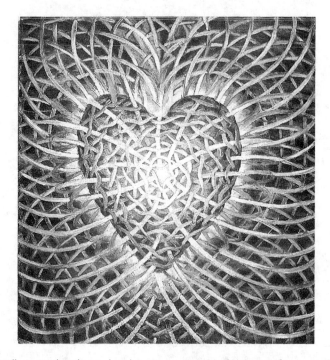

Nick Gadbois, *Grail*. Body, mind, and spirit are one. From the center of our open heart, we are connected to the life force that heals us. Nick says, "I have painted the threads of light that connect my heart with everyone and the whole world. In a vision, I saw that the universe sees everything."

A Story of Healing Cancer with Art and Imagery

Michael tells this story of a person he worked with.

A man came to see me who had metastatic liver cancer. The reason he came was to "let the energy that he knows is in him move from his center to the rest of his body." He felt he was blocked somehow and that sadness was keeping him from opening up to the world. Now this was an unusual chief complaint (that is what physicians call the answer to "Why are you here today?"). All chief complaints are new and different when you actually ask people what is on their mind and not just what illness they have, but this was not the response I would have expected from this type of person. He was a beautiful man, tall and gray haired and dignified. He was a wealthy businessman who had had all he wanted of the finer things in life. He had excellent taste and he surrounded himself with the best, and now he was very ill. His reason for coming was surprising to me considering how conservative a lifestyle he led. But it turned out he had gone to meditation classes for years and was deeply connected to his inner world.

When I first saw him, he made a sand tray of himself and his family. In a sand tray, you pick objects from a huge collection of miniature figures, animals, buildings, cars, and other things and arrange them in a tray of sand. The technique, which was pioneered by Carl Jung, is similar to making a painting or sculpture or even to telling a story. The man put the small figures representing him and his family in the sand, and he put down a toy house as his home, and up in the far right corner of the tray, he put a mystical figure that looked like nothing else in the sand tray and he made a sun ring around it. I asked him if he knew who this figure represented, for he had told me about all the other objects in the sculpture—but this one he had left out. He said he didn't know what the figure was and it puzzled him deeply. I closed my eyes and looked around him. I saw and felt a presence over his right shoulder. I asked him if he felt anything around him. He stopped and meditated and tears came into his eyes. He said that he saw a light and felt a warmth above him. I asked him to slow down time and to see in between the moments. His breathing became deeper and he suddenly sat up straight. "I see an angel, and she is so beautiful," he said.

"Do you recognize her?" I asked. His eyes were filled with tears.

"She is my daughter who was killed in an accident."

"Does she want to tell you anything?"

"She is pointing her finger at my liver and light is coming out of it and it is flowing into me. She is telling me that she is my angel and that she will help heal my cancer."

The next time I saw him he was deeply changed. He looked much more alive; he was full of energy and almost seemed to vibrate. He told me that the ground under his feet caressed him as he walked, the wind kissed his face, he walked at a slower pace, and he was at peace. He said that the earth sent healing energy up into him and that it tingled, that his morning walk was now enchanted. I asked him to tell me what the energy of the earth felt like. He told me that it was like tiny fireflies flying up into his body and making him feel more alive. It was like the earth was sending her love up into him. When he told me this, he cried. I asked him if the energy in his spine could now move all over. He told me it could. I helped him feel the flow of his energy when I moved it in his body with my hands and then with his. I often move my hands over people's bodies and have them feel energy move inside them.

One month later he called me to tell me that his liver scan had come back completely negative. The three large metastatic nodules that were growing and had been there for a year were now gone. Making the art in the sand tray showed us his angel. It would have been more difficult to see it with guided imagery alone, and much more difficult by any other means. Art is the best way for an ordinary person to see a transformative spiritual vision. Seeing the angel put him in the physiology of healing, where his immune system ate the cancer cells. I do not take responsibility for his healing himself of cancer. He was getting the best cancer care from an oncologist, he had changed his diet, he did his yoga, he had people praying for him, and he had put together a wonderful holistic cancer care regimen that included me and healing art. I believe that what he did as a person with cancer was right for him. Everyone can put together a "healing pie" that includes all the modalities he used or anything that feels good to them. Art can be a part of any person's healing force; it is the part that fills you with energy and changes your life.

This kind of story is why we do the kind of work that we do. I was allowed to be part of this man's intense beauty and share his light. I was allowed to see what he saw. I was allowed to be with him as he was healed. When I started out as a physician, I was taught that medicine involved doing what was proven by scientific studies. I had done immunogenetic research studying the white blood cell's ability to make antibodies against foreign substances, and I knew what a good research study was. But as I started seeing patients with cancer, the world I found myself in was much different from the world I had been taught to see. If I was to actually listen to the stories of the people I was seeing and respect and love them as human beings, I needed another worldview.

As I listened to their stories and saw them heal, I found that I had deep beliefs in a healer within that were not at that time supported by double-blind studies. At first I was in a dilemma. Should I wait for studies to be done on guided imagery before I did this kind of work with my patients? I could not. I knew imagery and art would not hurt them and that I would continue giving them the best allopathic care, but I also knew that my life was changed, that I had to do what I believed in—I had to make my own inner experiences part of my external world. At that time I started to do guided imagery with patients who wanted it. Many years later, studies were done that showed that imagery affected the immune system and blood flow. Finally there was patient data to support this therapy. I was glad I had used it for twenty years before the studies were done.

Art and healing is now in the same place in the progress of research that imagery was in twenty years ago. We know art heals, and yet we do not have many good randomized studies directly proving it. The studies are being done now. Basically the research is of two types: patient outcome studies and physiological studies. As these studies show us that art heals, it may be easier to fund art and healing programs that are starting in hospitals all across the country. However, there are many good studies already published that link art to reduced pain, that show that art improves the quality of life, that describe the impact of art on different patient populations and illnesses, that relate art and symptom relief, that connect art and attitude and empowerment, and yet these studies have not changed medical practice as much as they should have. Many studies showing that music reduces pain have not helped put music in every hospital. If a drug were found that was shown in studies to do what art does, it would be used extensively. Only the passion of a musician and a doctor or nurse working together has done that. It is only our beliefs and passions that cause change; it is only our love for this work that makes it happen.

THE PHYSIOLOGY OF ART AND HEALING

For the nurse or physician in the medical center, art and healing involves observing how thoughts, emotions, and images change blood flow and hormone balance in the body. As we make art, we see images. The images involve the firing of neurons in different areas of the brain. The firing neurons, the nets of cascading activity, connect to the body in three simple ways.

First, the right brain, the home of imagery, sends messages to the lower brain areas, which connect to the hypothalamus. Images of art, music, movement, and dance are initially held in areas that are responsible for thought and instituting muscle movement. The discharges of neurons come from both the making of art or doing a movement and the memory of art and movement. The way it feels to people is that a thought, an idea, or an image of art, music, and moving comes from their imagination or memory. Since art, music, and dance are so ancient and involve so many sensory and motor pathways, both the imagination and memory of art, music, and movement appear very real and intense as a person gets in touch with them. The movements are reflected as discharges in areas that send messages to muscles, and even if the artist or dancer does not actually move those muscles, they move microscopically.

The places where the images of movement are held send nerve messages to the hypothalamus that are processed and then go out to the rest of the body. Likewise, the image or dance movement itself is picked up by the brain, and that area sends messages to the hypothalamus. So the artist or dancer's brain sends out messages to the whole body if there is a movement, or even if there is an imagined movement. The areas of the brain that control movement have in them the memory of previous images or dance movements that are stored in memory pathways. I believe that many of these memories of images or movements are ancient, flickering steadfastly within the human brain as it evolved. When these visions come to the surface of our consciousness and are released, it can be deeply healing.

When a person translates images in the mind into art made by muscle movements, a deep level of concentration is produced. Making art takes the person's whole attention and takes the person away from the worries and concerns of the outer world. This happens automatically. The person does not need to do anything except make art to focus intensely. The ancient neural pathways of the mind take over and the person is taken "elsewhere" to a mental state of pure concentration that most resembles meditation. The physiology that results from this state is similar to the physiology of prayer and meditation and basically involves deep relaxation and healing. Dr. Herbert Benson at the Behavioral Medicine Clinic at Harvard University Medical School wrote about this in his classic *The Relaxation Response*. He showed that meditation alone lowered blood pressure, heart rate, and breathing rate and was a primary therapy for heart-disease patients. Today, Dr. Dean Ornish uses meditation as a major part of his heart-disease regimen to reduce stress. He also uses it for its spiritual focus to reduce alienation and promote feelings of connectedness and oneness.

How does this physiology process work? Images held in the right brain activate the hypothalamus. The hypothalamus activates the autonomic nervous system and results in arousal or relaxation of a double balancing system that impacts the whole body, touching virtually every cell. The autonomic nervous system is a healing system that balances and maintains the blood flow, heartbeat, breathing rate, and hormone level needed for any activity we are doing. It is also the system that we need to heal. This system was thought to work by itself, but it is now known to be profoundly influenced by thoughts in the mind. The autonomic nervous system has two branches, the sympathetic and the parasympathetic. The sympathetic branch of the auto-nomic nervous system is the branch that controls "fight and flight," creating the physiology necessary to run from a tiger or assume the defensive pos-ture. The image of a threat in the large hemispheres of the brain alerts the hypothalamus, causing sympathetic arousal, and this speeds up the heart-beat, increases breathing, sends blood to the large muscles, floods the body with adrenaline and stress hormones, and thus creates a physiology of alert-ness. The memory of running away from a threat or facing it and fighting and getting away takes us through a whole cycle of experience. When you are out of danger at last, the feeling of safety relieves tension and puts you in a state of release. The cycle is called the arousal/release cycle, and it charts each person's way of reacting to any exciting event.

On the other hand, the stimulation of the parasympathetic branch of the autonomic nervous system results in relaxation, in healing, in body repair, in preventive maintenance. The image in the brain of a peaceful scene, of making art, of creativity, of prayer, alerts the hypothalamus to trigger a parasympathetic arousal and the heartbeat slows, blood pressure drops, breathing slows, blood goes to the intestines—the whole body changes. The dance movement of a soft caress stimulates the circuits that remember deep relaxation and creates that physiology. We now have the physiology of healing, of creativity, and of prayer. This oversimplified model gives us an idea of how the mind is connected to the body and how images and muscle movements stimulate our entire being. When we picture art, music, or a dance movement, or make art or dance, the area of the cere-brum that holds images of muscle movement is stimulated, and it sends messages to the hypothalamus that allow us to respond to the imagery. If the image is one of deep joy or release of tension, our body is put in a healing state through the hypothalamic pathways of the parasympathetic nervous system. When the artist puts down an image of himself in pain and that vision is seen for the first time, the tension around the pain is felt and then released. Relaxation ensues and the healing physiology is started.

Second, we have the hormonal flood that bathes every cell in the body as the imagery of threat or passionate creativity lights up the neural nets in the brain. As the nerve cells discharge like a loom of light flashing through the brain, the hypothalamus sends messages to the adrenal glands to release epinephrine, adrenaline, and other hormones. These hormones travel throughout the body and are picked up by receptors that cause some cells to contract, others to relax, some to act, others to rest. So our entire physiology is changed a second time by an image or dance movement held in our brain, our consciousness. The second change is chemical, resulting from hormonal shifts. It is slower, but it is just as profound in that it affects almost every cell in the body.

Finally we enter the realm of the neurotransmitter. This is a third way art changes the body's physiology. Here, images cause specific areas of the brain itself to release endorphins and other neurotransmitters, which affect brain cells and cells of the immune system. The neurotransmitters relieve pain and make the immune system function more efficiently. They cause killer T cells to eat cancer cells and white blood cells to attack AIDS viruses and generally change the body's ability to respond to illness. So when a person makes art or music, or dances, or pictures an image that is freeing and joyful, the body actually changes its physiology to heal itself. The release of the endorphins when we make art is felt as deeply pleasurable. It is like a person exercising. The endorphins are like opiates or mind-altering drugs, and they make a person feel expanded, connected, at one, relaxed, vibrating, tingling, at peace. In a real sense, the release of endorphins during passionate creativity may be the major healing force. It is psychoneuroimmunology at its best. *Psychoneuroimmunology* is a term that puts together *psycho* for the mind, *neuro* for the nerve nets of the brain, and *immune* for the immune system to describe how thoughts or images in the mind affect the immune system. One artist we interviewed heard our question "How did you end up where you are?" as "How do you endorphin?" The concept of endorphin release is basic to the way she looks at art and healing.

So what do we have here? We are in the midst of a modern story or scientific theory that basically says that a thought, image, or muscle movement changes a cell and helps us heal. It does this in three steps: 1. A thought, image, dance movement, or piece of art is created; 2. a message is sent to the cells by a nerve impulse, a hormone, or a neurotransmitter; 3. the cells become activated, eating a cancer cell or virus, sending blood to an area of illness, or relaxing or tensing. This is a simple model. It is biolog-

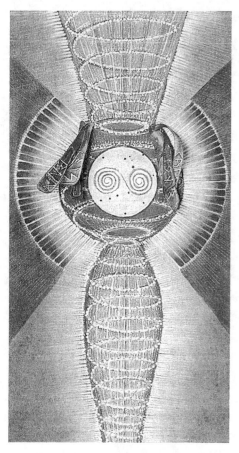

Barbara Bruch, *Spiral Goddess*. Healing energy has always been seen as spirals. We see it as coming from your artist within. "My work reflects my own spiritual journey. I think of my paintings as a shamanic force expressing healing experiences both for myself and for others on the spiritual path. During a meditation, one looks at the painting and thinks about the healing energy of the body and attempts to visually direct it to the afflicted area. Some pieces of my current work have been referred to as energy-healing paintings and meditational mandalas. Some of my paintings depict a moving healing energy in the use of color."

ical, physical. It tries to connect the mind and body, which it still sees as separate, but it at least sees them as speaking to each other. It does not view the body as an automaton uninfluenced by thoughts and perceptions or the mind as irrelevant.

The evolution of this model took half a century and was a great step forward in modern science. It defied the Cartesian split of mind and body that ruled science and even psychology for a century and prevented perceptions, emotions, and life experiences from entering medicine. When we went to medical school and nursing school in the sixties and seventies, we were still taught that the mind does not affect the body, but now, thankfully, that training is outmoded. Now we know that when your mind makes an image, or your body makes art, you produce the physiology of healing in every cell of the body, including the immune system.

NOW LET'S PUT IN THE SOUL

So, with this oversimplified three-step model in mind, let's drift gently back to the world of our experiences. How did that model make you feel? Safe, solid, bored, confused, science ignorant, grounded, cold, convinced, secure? It may not be spiritually elevating for me, but it is very useful, almost necessary, to understand as a base of belief, a connection between the worlds of science and the worlds of art. So let's drift back into art, let's feel again how art opens our hearts and relate that to the three-step model. Let's imagine making art with people with cancer, seeing them come into our studio with a beautiful child, seeing them paint, seeing them look into their babies' eyes and then trace the babies' hand over theirs and get tears in their eyes and feel love all around them. Just trying this for a moment tells us that there is something incomplete about the model of mind-body alone. As we close our eyes and feel our heart opening, as we watch our patients heal and feel their love, as we hear a song of love or see a dancer enter a hospital room or view artwork in our sacred space, our shrine of rebirth, the three-step model doesn't seem to tell us enough about our experience. It is not an accurate description of how much more we feel and see.

So here is another model, one that merges medicine with our spiritual beliefs, one that comes a little closer to describing how we actually feel inside. Remember, this too is just a scaffold, a structure to try to explain the ineffable, to try to put a foundation beneath us as we undertake the exciting journey of trying to understand how art heals.

We see our body's spirit attracting matter around it like a cloak. The spirit is more like what we see as our soul. The idea has no independent existence; it is of the whole. From far within, from the reaches of the deepest space, this idea has grown, formed, reformed, and changed. If you go deep into the darkness, far back, way back, downward, downward, you reach the place of birth. From there flows our soul, our spirit, the first manifestation of light. And from the darkness, wholeness, where there is no beginning or end, no time and little space, the soul grows, expands, and enters the mind and body for a while. And so body, mind, and spirit form an aggregate, an entity, a being. And that being is you and me, whole and one and at the same time connected.

The body's health depends on its balance, its physiology. When its systems are in order, blood flows at a certain pressure, the heart beats at a certain rate, the hormones are in a certain balance. Many of us now see this balance as coming from a dialogue of body, mind, and spirit. I see the spirit awakening, being awake, being listened to, talking to the mind and the body. It tells the mind and the body both through the body's feelings and tension levels and through the mind's feelings, emotions, images, and thoughts how to balance. When the spirit is not listened to, imbalance results. This feels like discomfort. When the spirit is listened to, the body, mind, and spirit resonate as one, the spirit dances and sings, and healing happens. The spirit dances itself to you, sings its song to you, paints its picture for you. And when the spirit becomes alive, the inner healer that is body and mind working as one is free. Gone are the tension and fear that block this healer when the spirit is asleep, and the blood can flow to a cancer, bringing with it the immune cells and natural chemicals and chemotherapy drugs that kill the tumor.

HOW ART HEALS

- Autonomic nervous system shifts the body to the relaxation response.
- Hormones shift the body to a healing mode.
- Blood flow shifts, bringing in nutrients and immune cells.
- Immune system enhancement fights cancer and infection.
- Killer T cells eat cancer cells.
- Neurotransmitters and endorphins reduce pain.
- Self-healing mechanisms are released.

MIND: SHIFT TO ONE-MINDEDNESS
- Focus and concentration take you "elsewhere."
- Attitude becomes hopeful.
- You experience feelings of peace and joy.
- Priorities shift to value life.
- Images of healing are released.

SPIRIT: AN EXPERIENCE OF TRANSCENDENCE
- You see God.
- Inner power is released.
- Images of spirits and helpers are seen.

SPIRIT AND THE INNER WORLD

When you ask artists about healing, they talk of light, of darkness, of places in the inner world where they see the visions for their paintings. They talk of how freeing their spirit helped them heal. They don't talk about white blood cells. Gordon Onslow Ford, a surrealist painter, has written about art and the inner world extensively. In his writings, he calls the places of creation within us "the deep spaces." He believes that the true haunt of the pioneer painter is the place of creation, the furthest inward one can go in the imagination and see creation. Only by doing that, he feels, can the artist see the truth and bring it out to share with us. We do the same process when we work with patients. Art takes them as far into their inner world as they want to go. So we have an experience of the inner world with patients similar to that which Gordon has with making art.

Gordon believes that far within us are the deep spaces, the furthest reaches of the soul. By traveling inward, we can glimpse worlds, feel them, live in them. And we can bring back their memory traces, bring back their spirit, only with art (by "art" we mean all the arts: painting, sculpture, storytelling, poetry, music, and dance). We believe that the voices of the inner worlds, of the spirit, speak to us in a language that is most comparable in our world to art. It is below words, it is above silence; it is closest to poetry, music, and dance. It is God singing and dancing. It is our soul listening. It is the voice within us of the life force, of expansion, of love. It is the connection, the real bridge, the source of all power.

And when we pray, when we travel inward and see, we can bring back traces of the pure spirit. These footprints are art. Art is the voice of the spirit. And when the spirit is freed, when the spirit is seen and heard, the inner healer is released.

HEALING ENERGY

And here we must speak of healing energy. When you talk of healing, when you experience healing, you feel energy. When we talk of a resonation of the body, mind, and spirit, we mean a freeing of energy, a buzzing, a tingling, a vibration, a hovering. And the energy is felt as a sensation, a feeling; it can flow throughout the body, from body to body, from the universe to us. It can be seen by psychics and meditators and can be portrayed in art. What is this energy? Chi, prana, kundalini, God's breath, acupuncture energy meridians, chakras, the life force? It has been described throughout all time. It is an integral part of the human experience. Because art acts at the level of the spirit, because art is the language of the spirit, energy is involved. Perhaps the simplest metaphor for how art heals is that it frees our body's healing energy to flow. This is the image of the Kalihari dancing in the previous chapter. The image is seen by the spirit; the spirit soars, goes home, unites with the deep source; and energy is released like a torrent, like a breakthrough, like a waterfall. The bringing home releases energy. That is all. The making of art puts you there by itself. You need not do anything except make art.

GUIDED IMAGERY

What are these things called images that we have been talking about and how are they related to art? Images are thoughts that come as imagined lived experiences. They have the shape of the sensory modalities that feed them. They are part of real time in that we feel them as touch, sound, sight, smell, muscle position, and taste. They are beyond real time in that they can glimpse realms that cannot be experienced with our ordinary senses.

Psychologists divide imagery into several categories. Memory images evoke events that took place in the past. Imagination images are not based on discrete events from the outer world; they are the result of combining memory events in new and creative ways or they come from outside us, from the world of the spirit. Dream images are experienced in sleep. Hypnopompic images are the visions we see as we awaken; hypnagogic images those we see while falling asleep. Visions are images experienced while awake or in a trance that are very vivid. Hallucinations are images experienced while awake that are poorly controllable. (*Vividness* and *controllability* are terms that show us how psychologists describe the imagery experience. When the experience of imagery is intense, when the images are bright, loud, or very attention-getting, they are "vivid." When images are unbidden, cannot be gotten rid of, or cannot be changed, they are "poorly controllable.")

In his book *Seeing with the Mind's Eye,* Michael divided imagery into two basic types—receptive and programmed. Receptive imagery comes to you; it arrives on the scene, bidden or unbidden, and rests in your mind's eye. Programmed imagery is different. You choose an image and hold it in your thoughts for a reason. The choice may be deliberate or you may choose an image that came to you from the receptive space. Either way, the image affects your world.

How do healers work with imagery? The most common technique involves having patients picture their illness, their healing forces, and the healing process in their mind's eye. First the patients imagine what the illness looks like in as much detail as they can. Next they imagine how the body's resources could deal with the visualized illness. This is imagined as a process over time. For example, patients can picture cancer cells, picture them in an area of the body, picture them as a certain color, shape, smell, texture. They then can picture killer cells or white blood cells eating the cancer cells and the body's defenses advancing, multiplying, engulfing the cells whole, and wiping them all out.

This biological imagery is more effective if it is anatomically accurate and detailed. Researchers have found that this imagery is very specific. For example, if one type of white blood cell is pictured, its blood count alone is found to rise. Next, patients are encouraged to allow metaphorical imagery to form. This is the stage where little men, dogs, or white light blasts, eats, or dissolves blackness, mud, or other little men. Generally, this metaphorical imagery takes place spontaneously after the biological imagery. Finally, patients can hold a programmed image in mind. They can picture themselves healed, surrounded by white light, surrounded by energy, as a God, as a power animal, or as strong and secure.

So healing art, like guided imagery, can be used by a patient in two obvious ways: the images can be viewed and the balancing nature of them can be allowed to change a person's consciousness, or images can be used to help a person visualize the healing process or a healed state. In both types of healing, the art provides imagery seen by the artist. The imagery is healing if it relaxes, allows release of tension or fear, puts people in an altered state, opens their heart, or moves them and gives them energy. Monet's *Water Lilies* was so relaxing that people with a wide range of illnesses would visit the museums and sit and meditate in front of the painting for hours. From the point of view of this model, the water lilies were memory images, rendered as art, evoking in the viewer a physiology of healing. The painting put the viewers in a state of deep relaxation, in the place of Monet's spirit, in the place of water, light, and color, in the place of intense beauty and harmony.

The third way art heals a viewer is by showing patients images that move them emotionally. When patients with breast cancer, for example, see art, music, or dance made by other breast cancer patients, they are opened up to emotions they may have hidden. This allows them to discuss these emotions with family, support people, and their healers. Patients who have a particular illness are moved by art that portrays other patients' experiences with the same illness. It makes them feel connected, relieves isolation, and releases deep emotions. This type of art can be very disturbing for other people to view. The images are often gory or graphic. This imagery is not for relaxation or transcendence; it is for opening the heart.

HEALING ART

For the healing artist, there are several types of healing art: relaxing, balancing images whose presence is transformative by itself; biological images that provide a library of images to visualize; and images of pain that are moving and result in a release of emotions. This last type of healing art provides a cathartic release, an emotional discharge. During disease or in any major life event, stress builds up. The stress can accumulate and get held in the body, lost inside hidden memories. Making art opens a Pandora's box of deeply held secrets. The art releases the stress like a dramatic explosion. The release causes your body to reachieve balance. All these types of healing art are powerful and effective. They all work by changing consciousness, by freeing energy, by awakening the spirit to resonate body, mind, and spirit. This is the technology of healing art, its tools, its machines.

Images made by artists can be so powerful, so filled with energy, that even though they are not personal to the patient, they too can be transformative. Throughout recorded history, artists have believed that their images have power in themselves. Shamanic art was believed to actually have the power to change the physical world. Its shape and color were believed to be powerful in themselves, to be able to transmit and move real energy. Just standing near a piece of healing art was believed to heal. No viewing was necessary, no understanding obligatory; it was just an experience that brought about molecular change. This concept is difficult for many Westerners to grasp scientifically, but it is not that foreign from our lives. People carry good-luck charms, relics, and holy objects; they make shrines, sacred spaces, churches, and meditation rooms. Patients surround themselves with power animals, religious talismans, and crystals. The belief in the healing energy of objects is deep, even in our rational, logical world.

A GUIDED IMAGERY EXERCISE OF THE OLD WOMAN OF THE SPRINGS: HOW SHE MADE OUR BODIES TO BE HEALED WITH ART

This chapter's story of the old woman of the springs relates how she made our bodies to be healed with art. She tells us that she made us with creative forces and that we are engaging in the same process when we make art. The old woman of the springs in this legend is the spirit mother. Many healing artists have told us that the new line they draw on a blank page feels the same to them as creating a new body to heal, making new healthy cells. It is creation; it is making something out of nothing. This is a story of how she made us of light and energy, as we make healing art of light and energy.

> Close your eyes. Go back to the springs; see the old woman of the springs sitting above you weaving. Listen to her story. She wants to talk to you now. Relax deeply; listen to her song. She sings to you, "I want to tell you how art heals, for I know that people have been taught that their bodies are made of only matter and energy. Do you see me sitting above the springs

looking down at you in perfect love? Do you see me now as a painter with my paper and paints? Look deep into the center of the springs, my child. See the water flowing upward from my blue white light, see it bubbling forever up from the light into the deep blue pool and then resting for a moment and then forming the river that flows crystal clear from my heart to the whole earth. And I sit above you both as the painter and the weaver, and as I paint the spirals in the spring, and as I paint the world, you can see the silver threads coming from my hands to the spring and the silver threads coming from my hands to the painting and the silver threads coming from above into me. I weave the tapestry of the world, of healing art. As I paint, the world comes into being. As I paint, the silver threads from above that are Her pure love, coming from before the beginning of time, from the place of peace, come into my body and into my eyes and into my hands. And as I put down a line or a circle or a dot, my body remembers Her dream as She made the earth. And as I paint, I again paint it all into being. The silver threads that come from Her into me go outward, and in my love and in my dream I weave them into the spring and into the waters and into you, my child, and into your body.

"And as I am the woman of the springs, the weaver of the earth, my art is the world. Watch me carefully, my child. Look at my fingertips. See the light coming from them in sacred spirals spinning outward. See the matter forming around the light dancing to it and popping from it and coming into being. As I weave the world, I weave your body. As I weave the world, I weave your inner healer, I weave your immune system, I weave your self-healing abilities, I weave your ability to heal. As I weave the universe, I also weave your bodies, for they are of the same fabric. They work in the same way. I weave your bones and muscles and blood vessels of the stuff of the stars. I weave your energy and your vibrations of the energy of the spheres. I weave your souls *and your spirits of the dreams of the ancient ones. I weave your heart and your love of the love that created the universe, of our mother's love. See the waters forming on the silver dots that flash as I move like fireflies in the night. See it all being born, as I love you out of my love and light. Do you not see it? Feel me touching you and feel your body being born anew and being born as a light body to be healed. How does art heal? As I paint the world into being and as I touch you with my dots of light that come from Her heart, you are made anew in my vision, as I am the creator and the manifestor of form. How does art heal? As I paint and touch you with my fingertips, I make my vision of pure love become matter; I dream the world into being and I make it as art and as matter at once. Can you do less? For you are me and I love you perfectly."*

THE PROOF THAT ART HEALS

When we go to conferences and talk about art and healing, people often ask us if research needs to be done to help art and healing be incorporated into health care. The question "Do we need scientific proof that art heals to use healing art?" is very much an issue with physicians and hospitals today. For us, the answer is simple. It is provided by our own body. To feel it, close your eyes a moment and try this brief guided imagery.

Relax; take several deep breaths; let your abdomen rise and fall as you breathe in and out. Now go into the space where you make healing art, the space where you heal yourself, someone else, or the planet . . . drift, spin, turn, whirl. . . . Go into the space where your imagery comes from, where your visions are born . . . imagine yourself listening to your favorite music or singing, watching a dancer or dancing, looking at a relaxing painting or painting. Imagine a wonderful artist is making art with you, for you. Go with the art, fly on Her love . . . let Her carry you into Her heart . . . deeply further and further . . . deeper and deeper. . . .

Feel Her love all around you; see His light surrounding you; feel it go into your heart and feel it flow into your soul. See the light come alive . . . see the images and come and make your art; feel yourself fly . . . feel yourself heal.

Do you need proof that you are an artist, that you are a seer? And yet we are always asked for the studies that prove that art heals, that it improves quality of life, cures illness, or lengthens life. This is very pertinent to people who are living with a life-threatening illness and are looking for ways to make themselves better or improve their life. And it plays a part in funding, implementing programs, motivating people to continue their work, and moving art and healing forward as a field both for artists and for healers.

Art as a complementary therapy is currently being studied in randomized research that is being done showing its effect on many physical and mental illnesses. Many studies show how art, music, and dance can improve quality of life, decrease pain, help attitude, relieve depression, and help symptoms disappear. But this is not the whole story. Mind-body interventions in general are difficult and expensive to study and are fairly new in modern medicine. These studies are not funded by drug companies or companies making surgical or electronic apparatuses that generate large profits for the companies or health-care facilities. The research is also difficult to do because art is different for everyone, and individual ways of creating are different. Research on inner states of consciousness is always harder to do in the traditional way of collecting data. Relaxation and imagery were not studied for years after they were widely used, and even now guided imagery has not been proven to cure cancer or lengthen life. Yet it is a major complementary therapy used in almost every cancer center. Currently there are no definitive studies that show that art by itself cures cancer or lengthens a person's life. But, like imagery, it is so obviously beneficial to people that it is used widely.

There is also an ongoing discussion in body-mind-spirit medicine about the difference between healing and curing. Sometimes it is not possible to cure an illness and prevent death, but it is possible to heal the person's whole life so he or she can be fulfilled and connected to life until death. This healing of a life is extremely beautiful and meaningful to the people who are ill and their family and friends. Art has been shown to increase quality of life so markedly that it heals, even if it does not always cure. After all, everyone cannot be cured all the time. There is a time to die that is part of nature. Sometimes we have to accept that healing is as important as curing, although the patients always want to be illness-free and survive.

Fortunately, there are studies in parallel fields whose results apply to both imagery and art and healing. Guided imagery, in fact, is closely related to art and healing in that its basic mechanism is mind-body intervention, and its way of acting is related to freeing imagery from the inner self, balances the mind-body interface, and resonates in the soul. Do we need proof that the soul exists to use that word, or that God exists to pray?

The two studies that have been most influential in this regard are David Spiegel's study at Stanford showing that women with metastatic breast cancer lived twice as long when they were in support groups than women without support, and Fawzy's study from UCLA that showed that people with melanoma lived longer and had fewer recurrences with ten hours of structured support and education. These two dramatic studies of life extension with relatively minimal mind-body interventions lead us to postulate that an involved intervention like an artist making art with a patient could be very beneficial. Art and healing uses the core concepts of support, release of fear, attitude change, and feeling connected. In fact, art and support groups have much in common. One way to look at art as healing is that it is a way of caring, a way of loving, a way of honoring.

ABOUT TIME AND SPACE AND HEALING

Physicist Irving Stein from the University of San Francisco has a new and somewhat unique theory of time and space. Because he is a quantum physicist, he does not believe in the older vision of matter and energy, or time and space, being separate. For quantum physicists, everything is interconnected. And like other quantum physicists, he believes that the observer affects the results of all experiments. When you are there to watch, you change the results. Like other quantum physicists, he also believes that the interconnection of all things goes from one end of the universe to the other. When a particle moves on one side of the universe, another particle on the other side of the universe moves simultaneously. When a butterfly flaps its wings in Thailand, something changes in New York. You can see that this worldview is different from the one held by an ordinary person. Most of us still hold Cartesian reality principles, which basically state that cause and effect are independent of the observer, that matter, energy, time, and space do not affect one another, and that when one thing moves, it has nothing to do with anything else. Now, this old worldview works most of the time, when objects are large and move slowly, but it does not work when they are the size of subatomic particles or when they move close to the speed of light. In these situations, the old view breaks down and no longer predicts what actually happens in the world. In the world of quantum physics, light bends as the observer moves, matter turns into energy, time changes as we move close to the speed of light, and particles affect every other particle.

For healing, the Cartesian reality is a dated paradigm to hold as our major worldview. Healing, like physics, simply does not always work in slow or large systems. In fact, nonordinary reality exists in the same place the quantum physics exists, and in the world of nonordinary reality, probability is very different. A miracle is simply an occurrence that has a low probability of occurring in ordinary reality and a higher probability of occurring in nonordinary reality. One of Cartesian realities' main tenets is that the mind and body are separate, and spirit is a different thing completely. Descartes had to formulate this theory to avoid persecution by the church in the dawn of science, but separateness is an outdated paradigm for modern physics and also for modern healing.

Back to the theory of Irving Stein. As a quantum physicist, he has postulated that time and space are like little particles. They have a beginning and an end—a length as it were—and then stop. And there is a break. And they start again. Now, if you think that is strange, he has also postulated that they are the same. A particle of time is the same as a particle of space. They are interchangeable. And if you think about it, which he certainly did, if time and space are the same and if they start and stop, there is no time and no space between particles.

So modern quantum physics has found nonordinary reality. Shamans have always said that there is a place where there is no time and space, where natural laws don't apply in the usual way. And that is the place of shamanic healing. That is the place of miracles. Irving Stein stops before that point. He does not theorize that you can get into or use the breaks between time and space. They are there, according to his theory, but that is as far as he goes. The shamans go much further. They say that if you stop the world, you can slip between the particles of time and space and fall into nontime and nonspace, and that is precisely the nonordinary world of healing. And what is the best way to fall in between time and space? Make art. For that is precisely what making art does. As any child who makes art will tell you, time seems to disappear when making art, and space is all confused, and when they make art they feel as if they are "elsewhere." And elsewhere for a person who is ill means diminished pain, fear, and symptoms and concentration on creativity. So maybe part of the physiology of art and healing is the physics of nontime and nonspace. Making art puts a person in between time and space, in a place where their laws don't apply in the same way, where you as the observer create reality and influence outcomes, and where all is interconnected. Just as prayer is a way of changing time, space, and matter, so is the making of a piece of art the creation of a new space-time continuum, where miracles have a larger probability of taking place.

Within the framework of art and healing, health is balance, harmony, and resonance; illness involves blockages, contraction, and destruction. When a person is out of balance, destruction occurs in their inner and outer world. Art is a constructive way of allowing energy to manifest without destroying one's self or others. It is the most ancient way of getting in touch with the healer within. We do not need to know the pathogenesis and etiology of illness in this method, for we are dealing with the transformation of energy into artistic forms.

The illness energy seeks change whatever its cause. Art spirals energy into the space of creativity and a process of transformation occurs, manifesting in tangible new forms. Something is not done to you, something comes out of you in a way that you can personally deal with. The art is real, the process is felt, the patients can feel themselves empowered, tapping into their inner strength from their visionary world. They create the very process that empowers them. Art is the physical process of being a creator. You feel this experience, you live the experience of creativity, you fall in love with who you are, you know who you are, you love yourself perfectly. When people are ill and get chemotherapy, they need to be able to find their inner healer so that they can participate in this process in this way. The art is their own expression of their healer; their art becomes their companion and the manifestation of their healing journey. The art enhances their immune system and creates a healing physiology.

So how does art heal? The scientific studies tell us that art heals by changing a person's body physiology and mental attitude. To review what we said above, the body's physiology changes from one of stress to one of deep relaxation, from one of fear to one of creativity and inspiration. Art and music put a person in a different brain wave pattern; art and music affect a person's autonomic nervous system, hormonal balance, and brain neurotransmitters. Art and music affect every cell in the body instantly to create a healing physiology that changes the immune system and blood flow to all the organs. Art and music also immediately change a person's perceptions of the world. They change attitude, emotional state, and pain perception. They create hope and positivity and they help people cope with difficulties. They transform a person's outlook and way of being in the world. Art and music take the fear and replace it with pleasure and security. Art, prayer, and healing take us into our inner world, the world of imagery and emotion, of visions and feelings. This journey inward to what used to be called "the spirit" or "soul" and now is called by science "the mind" is deeply healing. For healing comes to us from within: our own healing resources are freed to allow our immune system to operate optimally and that is always how we heal. We go inward on the creative spiral together through art, writing, dance, and music.

PART 2

HOW YOU CAN USE ART, WRITING, DANCE, AND MUSIC TO HEAL YOURSELF

| FIVE |

You Are
Already an Artist

This is the "how to" part of *Creative Healing.* Again, it is for anyone who is ill or in a life crisis and for any artist or healer who wants to heal others with art. The chapters in this part are meant to be practical and immediately useful. Say you are a woman recently diagnosed with breast cancer who has always wanted to paint. You have found this book on healing yourself with art, or someone who loves you has found it and given it to you, but there is no art and medicine program in the hospital you are going to for treatment. Or say you are a man with AIDS who has always wanted to write poetry, and there is no poet-in-residence in the outpatient clinic you go to. Or say you are an artist or healer and want to use your talents to heal others, and there is no art as healing program for you to participate in nearby. For all of you, this part of *Creative Healing* will try to substitute for your art and healing program by facilitating your making art, just as artists would when they came into your room and helped you heal yourself with art.

We will be your artist-in-residence in several ways. First, we will talk to you in the words of the artist-in-residence. We have interviewed painters, storytellers, poets, dancers, and musicians, and we will pass their advice and love on to you. We believe that the best way to heal yourself with art is to make art, and to do it now. Whether you want to heal yourself, heal another person, or heal the earth, the first step is the same: start making healing art. The way to heal with paint is to become a painter, to paint every day. The

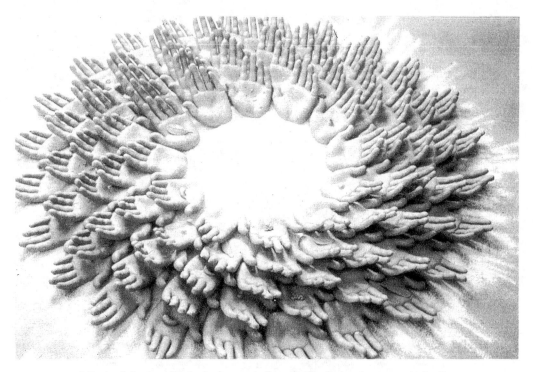

C. Regina Kelly, *Quan Yin*. Regina is an artist from Maine who has done extensive healing artwork in hospice. Her *Quan Yin* comes from the Japanese bodhisattva of wisdom who is often portrayed as a woman with a hundred or even a thousand hands. Each hand is holding a different remedy. With this, she can cure any illness. Each of the hundred hands on Regina's piece holds one of seven remedies: corn, stars, leaves, bear claws, eyes, flames, and flowers. She has synthesized curative nurturing symbols from diverse cultures into a universal symbol of compassion and healing. The artist is the gift giver. For many of us, this piece has become a beautiful symbol for the whole field of art and healing.

way to heal with poetry is to become a poet, to write a poem every day. This part of the book will empower you to do just that.

Making healing art is easy. Anyone can heal himself or herself with art. Through the work of our artists-in-residence, we have found that there are four simple steps to beginning. The first is to reclaim your inner artist. The second is to make a studio to create the space and time for yourself to heal. The third is to choose a medium that is natural for you. The fourth is to begin to make art with the subject that is the most meaningful and compelling in your own life. We believe that a book like this one is a tool. Like a hammer, it works in the physical world. It makes changes. With art, as with a wall you build in a new house, there is something to see at the end of each day. Your art is real and tangible; it can be seen, felt, or heard. Your healing will follow. Come, we invite you. Blessings, fellow artist healer, and welcome.

This part is not about teaching you how to make professional art. It is not an art lesson on how to draw or how to dance. It is instead an invitation to you to do whatever you want to do to explore what you are attracted to. In art and healing, the singing of one note can be as healing as singing a choral work. The writing of a paragraph as healing as writing a novel. The painting of a T-shirt for your child as healing as painting a masterpiece. We want to make the process of making art, dance, storytelling, and music as simple as possible so you can do it every day. All you need to do is give yourself a half hour a day. Whatever you choose to do needs to be as simple as possible so you can do it easily. Paint a half hour a day, write on a laptop a half hour a day, play the guitar a half hour a day. Maintain your creative work in a way that is easy and fun. That is what healing yourself with art is about. This "how to" section is not meant to be followed as a teaching of one method of making art. The road to get there will be your own. Any way you paint, write, dance, or make music is fine. In fact, to start out, the simplest way is probably the best. It will grow from there.

We have found that there is advice we can give you that works for all the media and is general enough not to hold you back. First, it is essential to be as flexible as possible. All the artists-in-residence always talk about being able to bend to the situation they find themselves in. If you are in bed and want to dance, you can still do it, you just have to move differently than if you were on a dance floor. Second, consistency is important in the beginning. Try to have enough consistency to make art every day. Know that this work is your gift to you to be healthy. You give yourself this time for you to be healthy, to feel alive, full, and as creative as you can. Value yourself enough to do it. Believe that this is simple and as important as anything else you do in life. In our culture, where most of us work long hours, this is about being free. We need a place in our lives and in ourselves to be truly free, to be who we are and to be ourselves.

THE FOUR STEPS TO CREATIVE HEALING

1. Reclaim your inner artist.
2. Make a studio: create space and time for yourself.
3. Choose a medium that is natural for you.
4. Begin to make art with the subject that is the most meaningful and compelling in your life.

THE GIFTS

When Mary healed herself with art, she set up an art program in the hospital. She had her artistic friend, who taught her to paint, become the first artist to work with patients and called her an artist-in-residence. Since the program started, there have been many artists-in-residence using all media. We will have the artists tell you their stories of how they have learned to make healing art. They are real people in real programs. The artists-in-residence who will speak to you in this part of the book are artists who believe deeply that art is a way of healing. They more than believe this; they live it with their whole lives. They are part of a community of artists all over the world who share this vision of art and healing as one. In fact, each artist has a gift to share with you. When we went around a circle of artist healers and asked them what gifts they would give you, the reader of this book, this is what they said:

"My gift is that you delight in your own essence and embrace the light of your spirit as it is reflected back to you from your own heart." Another said, "I am a gift giver, offering an escape into the creative world and its positive power of healing." Another said, "I will give you the pearl, the pearl of wisdom. Encourage your own self-expression, let yourself shine, let yourself be the star." Another said, "As an artist, I give the knowledge of what I know, and I am your servant. As an artist, I serve you by being kind and genuine. Although you will do art for yourself, you will only gain if you put others before you." Another said, "My gift is to allow the children I work with to still be children, to allow them to play, maintain the spirit of their child, while dealing with the illness." Another artist said, "The true gift as an artist is the goodwill and intention of bringing my gift to you. As we keep this in mind, all apprehension and anxiety will disappear." Open your heart and take your gift from the artists-in-residence. Pick one gift or more than one and take it for you. You deserve it. It is about loving you.

THE ARTIST'S GIFTS

- Delight in your own essence.
- Embrace the light of your spirit.
- Let yourself be the star.
- Allow the child to play.
- Intention is healing.
- The creative force is with you.
- It's only about loving you.

STEP ONE: RECLAIMING YOUR INNER ARTIST

Reclaiming your inner artist is one of the most important shifts you will ever make in your life. This process is about realizing that inherent in your life, inside of your life, is you as an artist. You have always been an artist, but you may not have seen it or valued it as much as you will now. This process is about illuminating the beauty within you. Our goal is for you to be able to say, "I am an artist" or, even better, "I am a healing artist." To internalize this concept, know that in everything that you do each day, there are opportunities to be creative. An artist is a way of being, a way of seeing. An artist looks deeply at light, at shadows. An artist looks deeply into each moment. The essential step is realizing that you want to be an artist. In most people's lives, there have been barriers and obstacles that have prevented them from doing it. Often this was due to a career choice or to criticism. Realize that all of us have had obstacles to passionate creativity. The obstacles will not hold you back anymore. In this situation, whatever it may be, it is worth the risk to become your inner artist now. Let go of any insecurities. The risk of your illness, depression, or lack of meaning in your life is more than what you feared in being an artist. This is an opportunity to let go of your fear.

What was threatening before is no longer important. When Mary started painting, she felt she was up against the wall, that there was nothing else she could do. The risk of not painting had become worse than the risk of painting. It was her time.

First reclaim the "Yes, I am an artist" that we all have within us. In the broadest sense, the definition of an artist is much wider than most of us think. We usually think that an artist is a painter, musician, dancer, or poet. But for healing art, an artist makes art in any and every way you can think of. We have separated ourselves from what we have done in our lives. We say we are not an artist as a mother, a physician, a gardener, whatever. We want to broaden artistry to include our whole lives. You can become clear that you are an artist in your work and in your whole life. It is a shift of who you think you are. Once a physician came to our workshops and felt awkward making clay figures. We told him he was an artist nevertheless. When we saw him next, he told us he realized what we meant. He realized he had in his medical practice the same feeling we talk about having when making art. He realized that he saw each of his patients with beauty. He saw them as interesting and their lives as precious. He treated them with care and even reverence. He knew he was an artist in the art of healing. When you reclaim your inner artist, you realize that there is an aspect of yourself that you illuminate like an artist. You reclaim a way of being that has been reserved for artists.

RECLAIMING YOUR INNER ARTIST

- Realize you want to be an artist.
- Let go of insecurities.
- Let go of fear.
- Say to yourself, "I am an artist."
- Broaden artistry to include your whole life.
- Realize that being an artist is natural.

A GUIDED IMAGERY EXERCISE: RECLAIMING YOUR INNER ARTIST

We believe that reclaiming the inner artist is the same natural process as the trees opening up each spring. Here is an imagery exercise that lets you feel how the tree feels as its new leaves emerge on that first warm day. As naturally as the leaves pop out of the branches, you will emerge from yourself as your inner artist. This guided imagery is to let you feel how natural making healing art is.

Close your eyes and relax; let your breathing slow and imagine yourself in the physical form of the tree. Imagine yourself as a tree, a tree growing from the earth. Imagine that the tree is the form of your being—it is your body; it is your physical experience. This is where your self resides. Imagine that as the tree, you have sensations, thoughts, and emotions. The tree is your ability to sense the world and your being within it. The tree is your being grounded in your life. Imagine that you are deeply rooted in the earth, that you are one with the earth and you are the earth at once. You are deeply aware of how you are connected to the earth and your environment. Imagine that you rest and grow and that the rain comes up inside you as the food. You are connected to the body of the earth like a tree is connected to the ground. Rest a moment and become aware of how you are deeply connected to the earth and your environment.

Now imagine that it is the first warm day of spring. The gentle wind blows through your branches; the sun warms your body. Be aware that you are from the earth and in the center of your body is a sap flowing. The sap is the sweetness of your own creativity. Feel the sap rising, feel it moving in a spiral up your body. See that inside your body is a sacred spiral that spins you into the being of your life. In this sacred spiral inside you is the central life force that spirals you into expansion and contraction along the space-time continuum of your life. Imagine that this eternal energy that spirals within you is a snake. This snake is a life force, it is part of you, it is not a snake from outside; it will not bite you, you are perfectly safe with it. Imagine that the snake spirals up from the earth that you are rooted in, up the trunk of the tree in your own body. Now imagine that in the very center of this spiral you can feel your heart. And now see that in the very center of your heart is an eye that is closed like your eyes are when you are sleeping. The heart is the center of yourself. It is the way you go inside the place of pure love inside yourself. The most important step you need to take is to open the eye in the center of your heart. When you open this heart's eye, you will see the world with love. You can see that you exist in the world; you wake up and begin to sense yourself and witness your own life. Imagine now that the eye in the center of your heart opens, and as you open up your eye, you can see for yourself.

Now let your arms be like branches on the tree and let them reach up toward the sky. The branches of the tree, as they reach up to the sky, follow your desire to reach up to the light. Your branches are the passageways of your energy up from within to the outside. Now imagine that there are tiny new leaves within each branch of your body. These beautiful new leaves are curled up under your skin or bark; they rest, waiting to come out into the light. You can't see your leaves from the outside until they open out, but each leaf is alive inside your branches. You know that at the right time they are born, and at the right time they fall to the ground. You know there is a creative process in each new light green leaf. Now imagine that each of your leaves comes out of the tree and into the world. They are physical manifestations of what is inside. They are manifestations of your being and the open eye within you. Now imagine that the leaves pop open into the light. One moment your arms are bare, the next they are covered with beautiful light green leaves. And each leaf is a story of the life of the tree, a story of your life now.

Each leaf is a poem, a drawing, a dance. Each leaf moves in the wind; each life is like a conversation with the world. Each leaf is your presence, a gesture, a creative act. Each leaf is a reflection of what has emerged from within you. Each leaf is your hand reaching up to the sky. See the new leaves as staggeringly beautiful. They are tiny, curled, almost wet in their newborn essence. But they are open and they can see the sun.

Now open your heart; open your eyes; open your leaves. Move with the tree; open your inner eye in the center of your heart. Be an artist. Let your leaves open as your art. You know the first bud that comes out of your body on the first warm day of spring as you begin to blossom and reach up to the sun? That same energy of renewal and rebirth is there for you as you become your artist, for you have seasons and cycles, too. In the most difficult of times, there is the moment of your recovery, the moment your leaves open, the moment you are an artist for the first time. Open your leaves now. Open your leaves now.

STEP TWO: MAKING YOUR OWN STUDIO

One of the most essential parts of the process of healing yourself with art is to allow yourself to create space to make art in your busy life. One of the ways you do this is by making a studio. Your studio can be a pad of paper, a laptop computer, a corner of the kitchen, a whole room at home, or a room out of your house. To make healing art, you make a commitment. You decide that your art is as important as anything else that you do in your life. It is as important as your children, your job, your lists, and shopping. It is as important as the most important thing you do, for making art is what will heal you, and your studio will be the space that you will go to to survive and heal. It is about finding an opportunity for yourself to do exactly what you want and need for yourself.

For many people, taking care of themselves is a crucial step. This is especially true for women who care for everyone around them. The decision to make yourself the focus of your healing process is critical. Making healing art is about you healing your life. When you do this, your family, children, and friends will be taken care of because you will be whole. You deserve it ... you do.

One woman who was a healer felt that she was selfish when she made her art. She was so used to taking care of others that when she gave some pure time to herself, she felt guilty. Then she realized that she had breast cancer and she deserved to be taken care of by others now and, more important, to finally take care of herself. So she made a piece of art with a healing artist that showed all the hands of all the people who were taking care of her, with a message of love to her to get well in each palm. It made her cry every time she read the messages and realized she needed and deserved the wonderful care her friends, family, and caregivers were giving her. A crucial part of her art was accepting that she as the caregiver needed and wanted to be cared for.

MAKING THE STUDIO BEAUTIFUL AND YOURS

The studio is the place where you will enter your passionate creativity. It is your doorway, your entryway. So make it the space where you will be the most comfortable. Put in personal things; find things you love and associate memories with, sacred things, beautiful things. Own it, for it is deeply yours. Pick a place with the light that you love, with music, favorite pens, photos, paintings, objects you are attracted to. You create these spaces, these conveniences, so that the artistic process is accessible, so you have inner privacy. Mary tells us more of her own experience:

> When I made my space, my friend Lee Ann helped me. I did not know what to do, I had never made a studio before. I had made houses for my family but never a place for me to be creative, a personal place. We brought in an old favorite rug. I put paintings I had done on the walls to remind me I could paint. I carved out a personal place, something I could move in to. We went to an art supply store and we just bought things. We bought paints,

brushes. Neither of us had done oils, and we did not know what to buy. We just grabbed things off the shelves that seemed to make sense.

You need to create a structure you can go into. You need a place to start from. An easel, blank paper, and water paints have to be right there so you can start to work. The empty blankness is an invitation to fill it up. Have enough room psychically and emotionally so you can daydream. Remember, it is about getting in touch with yourself, being in your own body, thoughts, and emotions. You take yourself out of the formal structure of your life. You make a void in the middle of it so you can use your own life as your palette. You need to put your life aside enough to look at it so you can participate in your imagery. You get a distance away to see yourself as who you are.

MAKING A STUDIO

- Create space in your busy life.
- Make a commitment.
- Regard art as the most important thing you do to heal yourself.
- Make yourself the focus of your healing process.
- Make the studio beautiful.
- Put personal things in the studio to make it deeply yours.
- Make the studio convenient and accessible.
- Create a routine to make art every day.
- Give yourself attention and listen to yourself.
- Create a boundary around yourself.
- Create sacred space with a prayer or altar.

CREATING A TIME TO MAKE ART

Every day create a routine. Work so many hours a day, or so many hours a week. But most important, create sacred time, a time undiluted by time as you ordinarily know it. Time is the most precious resource you have. When you give yourself time, it is the most useful gift for healing art that you can give yourself. You give yourself attention, you listen to yourself. In the studio, you can share with others, but you need your own space. You create a boundary around yourself—walls or rugs or bookcases—and you go into that place and work. At home, TV and your ordinary life keep you from it. This is an opportunity to go into your own world. You take a deep breath, and you go into a different flow of time and consciousness, a suspension of time. It is an experience of time that is different from everyday time. It has to do with being totally focused. You have to go in to be focused, for images to emerge. It is like giving birth—you pay total attention to what you are doing. In ordinary life you never are focused enough to be still, to go inward enough to be truly creative. The distractions are not healing. We go to a therapist to focus on ourselves, but this does it better. The focus and concentration create the physiology of healing and help the immune system function at its best.

Building a studio is like a bird building a nest in the spring. When the bird builds the nest, there are no babies, no eggs, only the anticipation of something about to be born. Build your studio like a nest, in anticipation of the birth of yourself as a healing artist. The eggs will grow and mature and one day there will be a baby bird. An artist makes or rents the studio, then starts painting, writing, dancing, or making music. The first attempts may not be much to look at, but they are important. One day the first healing painting will be born, one day the first healing poem or song or dance. Some people can create a process before the space. Everyone is different.

In another vision, a woman with a busy life does make art at home. She builds the studio in her life as a moment of time. She is creating a space in a different way. She goes in the kitchen for a half hour to write before everyone wakes up or before she goes to bed after everyone is asleep. In the same way, you can create this space—some people need a studio away from home, some people can work at home. It is organic; each person is different.

It is really about creating moments that are your own. Create a space right now in the moment. It is a conscious act that is deliberate, that has a space and a time. The space is sacred because it is the work of your heart, the work of who you really are. Dream of a space that is secret, like a wish to take you into a place in yourself where your heart is free. Make art with letters you never mail. Steal a moment to sing a lullaby to yourself, to another. Activate the artist within.

CREATING SACRED SPACE

Sacred space is really as simple as making meaning. A rock in the road does not mean much by itself; it is seen as something to sweep away. If you collected rocks, it could be precious if you needed it for your collection or if it were rare. If it were the rock that someone you loved had touched, its meaning would increase even more. If it were the rock that a holy person you revered had touched, it could be seen as deeply sacred. If it were the rock that Jesus or Buddha had touched before their death or as they were enlightened, it would be seen as sacred to a whole culture. Sacredness comes from the meaning in your life story. If you want to make art with intent to heal, make a space and a time that is full of meaning to you. The space you carve out of your life is the place where magic will happen, the place where you will be healed, grow, and change. It is as sacred as a church or mountaintop where you would receive a vision, for, after all, that is exactly what will happen. And the time, too, is sacred. This is a time that is only for you to do what you want to heal. It is a time of life and rebirth. It is sacred in its healing intent.

Many artists and healers make the space they work in sacred with intent. They stop for a moment before entering the space and say to themselves that the work they are about to do is sacred, full of meaning, full of life, holy, about life and death, about the spirits, about forces, about service, whatever way of looking at it that is their own story. One woman oncologist stops before entering each patient's room and prays, and imagines that the doorway is an arch as in a church, and that she is entering a holy place full of luminosity. And then she goes in, centered, and is a physician. Many artists who work with patients or make healing art in a studio say a prayer or do a guided imagery before starting work. The prayer is to make their work holy or full or rich, whatever they wish, and to make the space full of energy to allow the work to happen. Many people call in imaginary helpers or spirits or ancestors or teachers to help them. They do this in an imagery exercise or an intentional prayer. Many artists we work with have a whole ritual they do each time they make healing art or work with patients. They center themselves, quiet themselves down, pray to the helpers around them, whoever they are, and only then make art. So many healing artists do this that we look at it now as a part of the process of making healing art. That is the way it was done in ancient times, or with Buddhist artists. That is, in fact, the tradition we work from as healing artists. So before you make healing art yourself, consider pausing, centering yourself, and saying a prayer of healing intent to heal yourself, others, or the earth.

STEP THREE: CHOOSING A MEDIUM

When we have a physical illness, a depression, or a life crisis, or when we need to grow, we start to heal ourselves with art by opening ourselves up to our inner voices of change and creativity. We allow ourselves to listen to those voices and to let their messages to us emerge. In this process, choosing a medium is the next priority. Resonating with the medium is resonating with the creative process. Resonating means doing a type of artistic process that will flow with your energy. What is it that you do that flows with your body's energy? Everyone has different affinities for different types of art and different processes. You do not need to worry much about which medium you will choose, because when creativity flows it becomes multimedia, but you do need to start with something as the doorway, something that will allow you to have the sense of being an artist, so you can say, "I am a painter." Then the world will expand to other media.

When you use art to heal, you don't package the experience in one media, because it is not about making art to make art. It is more about making art to free yourself, making art to heal. When we talk about resonating with a material, the process is unique and personal for each individual.

Explore materials in the next chapters; read on and see what appeals to you. We will talk about many media. For example, in the chapter about painting we will discuss the difference between watercolors and oils. As you read, let yourself imagine doing it and see what you like, imagine how you would feel. Listen to the stories of the artist and how they work, and see if one of the stories feels like yours.

CHOOSING A MEDIUM

- Don't worry about which medium you choose.
- Remember a time when you were most creative as a child. Which medium did you use?
- Which medium resonates with your flow of energy?
- Which material comes to your mind first?
- Which process comes to your mind first?
- What is your secret desire?
- Allow yourself to experiment.
- Be open to choices ahead.
- Choose one.

There are two ways you see yourself as an inner artist: in the spirit world and in the real world. One is a dream, the other more practical. In the spirit world, Mary saw herself as a dancer, but in the real world she saw herself as a painter. Sometimes the real one is just easier, and your spirit world will follow as you learn to use many media. Or you may have chosen your medium already. You may have made art or played music before, or seen yourself as making art in your daydreams. Or you may have to ask yourself what you want to do. Am I a painter, a sculptor, a musician, a poet, a storyteller, a dancer? Have I ever wanted to create something but been afraid or too busy to do it? The artist is all of these people; the artist uses all media as healing.

To choose your medium, be open to the choices ahead. As you read the next chapters, don't be held to one and don't worry about which one to choose. Be confident that you will choose the right one. For now, don't close off any medium. To start to make a choice, go back in your life to where you were the most happy, or go back to a time in your life when you were doing something where you were most at peace. Go back in your life and examine that moment deeply. What surrounded you? What were you doing, seeing, smelling? Or go back in your life to where you were the darkest. What did you do to recover on your own? For example, if you were depressed as a teenager and you found you always went to the art school and worked on a dance project, that is a good place to start. When you were a child, did you write, draw, dance? As a child, you were more playful in problem solving, so go back and remember the circumstances and bring them up to your consciousness. Also, when you were a child, what did you always want to do? Did you want to be an artist, a movie star, a dancer? What did you want to do when you grew up? What did you want when you had no inhibitions, when you thought you could do anything and not fail, before you were hindered by life, when it was still a dream?

When you close your eyes, what one medium emerges for you? There are two times in your life when you were most likely to have been an artist: first as a very young child, next as a teenager. As a young child, you may have had art lessons or done art in school. As a teenager starting to separate from your parents to form your own identity, there were things you did naturally to become yourself. There is something from that place of individuation that can help you now. Go to what you were before you became an adult, before you became formed and more defined in roles. We will do an imagery to go back to both of those places, to see what medium resonates with us. But we will see more than that. We will see ourselves as artists again.

Mary tells her story:

I remember a moment in an art project when I knew I wanted to be an artist. I was an adolescent in a crisis. I was depressed and a runaway. At school, I went to the art room, not to other classes. The teacher would stare at me because I would never leave. I would add red color to the plaster to make the plaster pink. I was the only one doing that. I loved it. My teacher said it was wild, but in that moment where I was trying to be who I was, art was one of the only places I could rebel and not hurt myself or others.

Michael tells his story:

For me, it was painting an airplane mural in class. It was second grade. I had just moved. I had no friends and I stood and painted for days. It was the clearest space for me, with the least worry and fear.

A GUIDED IMAGERY EXERCISE FOR CHOOSING A MEDIUM

Close your eyes; rest; let your breathing get deeper; let your abdomen rise and fall as you breathe; let your body take over and take you deeper. Now go back to the moment in your life where you were a child making art. Go back in time through the past; go back many years to a point in your childhood where you remember a moment of making art that was full of happiness, a moment of making art where you were the most free. Go back to that moment in your life where you actually lived making art, where you allowed yourself to be truly creative and satisfied. Go back to that moment and go into your body. Remember how it felt; remember the world around you, the way you experienced the situation you were in, and spend some time in your child's body and be with that child. Be in the situation where you were making art as a child and watch your hands. Remember your thoughts. What did it feel like? And look at what materials you were using, and feel how they felt and how you felt, and totally be with it. Spend some time being with the activities you were doing. Feel your hands; feel your body as you were doing it. Be there and rest in its beauty.

Then go back to a moment in your life when you were in trouble, where you were sad or lonely or lost or upset. Maybe it was a time when you were a teenager, newly exploring who you were to separate from your parents. Go back to a time when you were discovering who you were. Go back to a moment where you were in conflict and pain, where you experienced despair. Go back to the darkness there; experience your full range of emotions and remember what you reached for when you reached into yourself. Remember who you were then, what you were thinking, what you were seeing with your eyes. Remember what you talked about, what you wanted to achieve. Was it writing poetry, making sculpture, painting? How did you explore the possibilities in your life? What did you do to get away from the problems, to go deep into your privacy, into yourself? Go to that moment, see what you were striving for. What were your desires?

Now remember a time in your youth when you were still uninhibited. What was that dream? What was the dream before life became so formed, when you thought anything was still possible, without any concept of failing? What was it? What were your dreams and desires, what was the glimmer of what you might resonate with, what did you do to go elsewhere and find out who you were? When you see yourself in a time of trouble, before you return, come back into the brightest place you know now in your life. Come back into the most beautiful vision that you can remember, a moment of love and joy. Let that moment of happiness wash over the moments of sadness from your past. Let them be cleaned; let yourself come out into the light and rest there now. Don't stay in the sadness after seeing it; come back now into your joy.

Next you will pick a medium, but the opportunity to integrate all the media in the process is important. We don't want to segregate the arts, to compartmentalize them into painting, music and dance, and poetry and storytelling when in our experience it is a more integrated process. We have found that being a healing artist is about being open to all the modalities. We separate them in the beginning because it's usually one medium you choose, but we have found it is an integration that actually occurs. The dancer, for example, uses all of the arts. In many programs, we've watched healing artists as they have evolved into renaissance artists. They walk into patients' rooms and can draw, dance, and even play music. They may be best at their own medium, but the rest come forth and make them more alive.

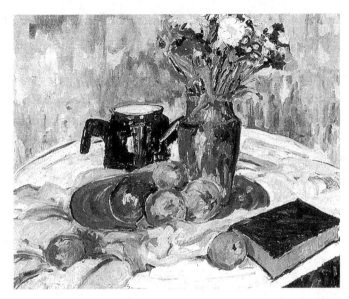

Mary Rockwood Lane, *Still Life*. Start painting from your own life. It is as simple as painting what you love, like flowers in your favorite vase with your most cherished book.

STEP FOUR: MAKING ART STARTING FROM WHERE YOU ARE IN YOUR LIFE RIGHT NOW

Finally, we make art. Next is the process itself—to draw, to move, to write or start a song. It is really simple, as simple as breathing or being in love. The experience of art and healing can be visualized as taking place on four spirals: the spiral of lived experience, the spiral of transformation, the spiral of empowerment, and the spiral of love. This description of how art and healing takes place is not theoretical; it is real. It comes from the experiences of people who have healed themselves with art, music, and dance, and it is taken from the actual stories they have told us. It starts from right where you are now. The first spiral of lived experience starts from your illness, your depression, your problems, your joy. The four spirals of art and healing are about you starting out from your life, about making the first piece of art simply from who you are now. We think the four spirals are useful because this way of seeing art and healing divides the process into four parts that you can look at separately. Its framework helps you to understand that the process is easy and automatic and yet powerful and profound.

The entire healing process can be pictured in your mind's eye in metaphorical form as a journey on a sacred spiral. The spiral down can be imagined as a concentric pathway of creativity. Spirals are concentric forces that bring people down into their own inner creative energy. When we reach the center of these spirals, we will reach the center of our heart where we are deeply connected to the world. Within the center of the heart, an inner eye opens up, the eye of awareness and witness. From the center of our spirit, we experience our inner connectedness. As the art comes out, you see that everything comes out, and that you are like everything. This is about birth. The art is what you are giving birth to. The art in this sense is an offering that heals you, an offering directly from your heart.

STARTING TO MAKE ART:
THE FOUR SPIRALS OF CREATIVE HEALING

THE SPIRAL OF LIVED EXPERIENCE
+ Make art with the stories of your own life, your illness, your experiences.
+ Go into your feelings and dreams, how your body feels, and your memories.
+ Move into your own experience.

THE SPIRAL OF TRANSFORMATION
+ Be in the moment.
+ Let inner wisdom emerge.
+ You are your own witness.
+ Make no judgments or criticism.
+ Allow your art to form.
+ Your art is a reflection.
+ See that you are changing.

THE SPIRAL OF EMPOWERMENT

+ Set your healer free.
+ Immerse yourself in the process.
+ Tap into your inner resources.
+ Feel your creative passionate fire emerge.
+ Look for signs of your power and strength in your art.

THE SPIRAL OF LOVE

+ Have faith in what is happening.
+ Be open to yourself.
+ Share your art with others.
+ Surrender to the process.
+ Bring forth your art as an act of love.

The Spiral of Lived Experience

The first spiral is the spiral of lived experience. The first art you make takes its subject from your life as it is now. You do not need to change to start, to be someone else, to pretend. You start from who you are now, from where you are now. This spiral is the spiral of your life—where you come from, who you are. This spiral comes from all of your stories of living, both beautiful and painful. It is the first meeting—where your eyes meet—when you see yourself, when you feel the events of your life. It informs you. It is about the experience of your life, your divorce, your children, your illness, cancer. It is what life has given you to work with, the material of your process. It is not an accident; it is the embodiment of your life, your thoughts, your emotions, your body—the embodiment of the experience of living. The actual pain and suffering is the palette, what you will use to make art, how you will discover who you are. The reality of living informs you in every moment of your love.

When you deal with art with the intention to heal, you deal with your own life. It doesn't come from books, from art school; it comes from who you are. In the beginning, you go into your life, you look at who you are. In the act of creating, there is movement and change, a technique, a process. The movement is inherent in the process. You become absorbed.

You go beyond your life into another space, into another world. Your intuitive nature—who you are—comes out. It is as if something else writes the story. There is confidence in an essential experience; it is tangible. There is the act of creation.

So as you make your first piece of art, come into the first spiral, into your feelings, dreams, into how your body feels, your ordinary memories, your emotions, body memories, how you are embodied in the world. It can be deep joy, deep pain, your cancer, depression. Go into the place where your tumor lies. Don't be afraid, for the spiral starts going in a circle, then goes inward toward your center, then starts again to spiral you into your light. You go into the place where you are in love again and it fills with fire. The event becomes alive again, not a memory of the past. You go into that space. You make a choice to take that energy that is inside of you, to take that energy and go deeper in the spiral. You do not have to think of a subject. In healing art it is there, it is you.

The Spiral of Transformation

The spiral of transformation is about art changing you. On this second spiral, you are making something, creating something. As you immerse yourself in your art, your consciousness expands and you may move to a deeper place, where you begin to glimpse yourself as beautiful and the wise person within you comes out. If you don't judge yourself, the beauty in yourself unfolds. You just let it come out when you go into that other world, and you see that your art is where you are, and where you were. You are now changing. The you that sees your art unfold is different from the you that was living in fear and unable to act. You look at the painting or read the journal and you see that you were like that, and now you are different. You are a person looking at a person who was. You are now changing. And you can see that the art is changing, too. The person and his or her worldview is new. You are transformed.

The Spiral of Empowerment

The third spiral, the spiral of empowerment, is about immersing yourself in the process. This is when you paint or make poetry in a passion. This is when

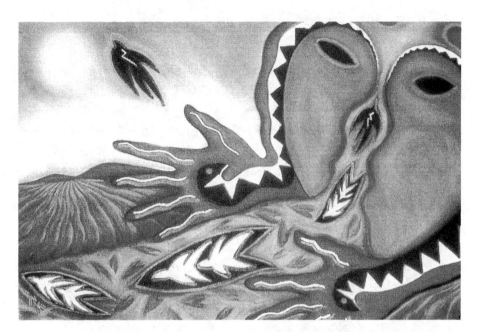

Julie Higgins, *Spillway from the Heart*. As we give, our heart overflows, and we share our art with the others around us. Julie says, "I believe in telling a story with my work, and therefore my work has evolved into a language of symbols. I work primarily with pastel due to its vibrant color and tactile quality. I work very intuitively with the color and forms—one image or symbol leading to the next. Heart images appear throughout my paintings; they are healing symbols for those transitions through life that recall pain and loss, and also hope for myself and the planet."

you are deep in the artistic process. In this space, you get to go elsewhere, into places where you may not be able to be in your life, especially if you are ill. You get to be who you want to be there. The process deepens by allowing you to experience your journey, to go from one place to another. The process is very tangible. It involves a mobilization of inner resources. This is where you tap into the passionate creative fire, a point of departure occurs, you immerse yourself into the creative process, and there is an experience of generation. Your inner strength and innate wisdom emerge. With no judgment, you can play and be who you are.

Then you go into technique, into process. You can paint, make music, do movement. With your feelings, you create a process to channel the love energy into a work of art. You go into the studio, you journal, you set aside time so that you fill it with that experience. You make a space in the world. You capture the experience in the present moment and make art from your body, thoughts, feelings. Something unexpected will emerge when you spontaneously let your body be what it wants to be, when you set the artist/medicine man/healer free. It can be painful. You can connect to your despair and your passion. In the hand of the artist, you have given it to Her; the artist heals by transformation itself.

The Spiral of Love

In the final spiral you are in love. It is about the art flowing from you like a spring, about giving your art away. You go to the place where you know who you are and accept who you are. You know yourself better. You know what your problems are and you accept them and yourself. You can deal with your life and create it as art in your life. This state of openness to the universe, to other people, to your own crises becomes your teacher.

SIX

Healing Yourself with the Visual Arts: Painting, Sculpture, Photography, and Crafts

Consider this an extraordinary journey we are about to take together. In this part of *Creative Healing* we will introduce to you to the artists and people who have healed themselves with art. These artists will act as guides and be your personal artist-in-residence. Their commitment is to share their creativity and support you in your own creative healing. Their intention is to fill your creative process with light and joy. Their years of experience will flow into you and remind you to reclaim your inner artist.

INTRODUCING YOUR PAINTER-IN-RESIDENCE

Welcome to my studio. My name is Mary Lisa. I am the painter-in-residence with the art program here. I am here to make art with you. If you are sick, or a family member of someone who is ill, or an artist who wants to learn how to make healing art with another person, I am here to show you how to do it. I am a visual artist, a fabric painter, a painter. I have been an artist since I was a small child. I have worked with patients in the hospital since 1993, and I will share this experience with you. I am your artist-in-residence today. What do you want to do? Let's put out a big piece of paper to make a body tracing. Let's put out a T-shirt with a pattern on it. Let's put out a piece of puzzle jewelry you can paint. Let's make a mandala circle painting of imagery you have had. Let's start making art.

Mary Lisa Kitakis is the painter-in-residence at the Shands Hospital Arts In Medicine program at the University of Florida, Gainesville. When you meet Mary Lisa, her eyes are sparkling, as always. She usually giggles as she is talking. At first she seems chatty, but when you watch her she hesitates to give you a chance to wonder what she is up to. Actually, it is like a tease. She is holding out the art supplies, getting everyone to play with her. Her brown hair softly caresses her face and is held up with a jeweled comb. She is always wearing something delightful with animals on it and many jeweled stars or rainbows. You know that what she will do will always be fun. She often sings as she moves and asks, "Does anybody want to play?"

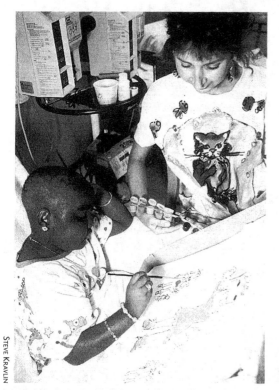

Mary Lisa Kitakis Painting with a Patient. Mary Lisa heals by encouraging us to return to the imagination in the child within.

HOW VISUAL ARTS HEAL

Visual arts have an immediacy of imagery that makes them the first doorway for many people who want to use art to heal. The first artists at the bedside in most hospital programs were visual artists. That may be because images of healing that come from deep in inner space often come up as visual images. Or it may be because there are more visual artists than poets or dancers who do this work. Visual images are more concrete than movement or sound, and for many people starting out, easier to connect with.

We constantly experience visual imagery in our lives, from movies and television to photographs, paintings, and sculpture. The concept of artist is tied to one who makes visual images. The first art most people think of is painting, and the first recorded art is the ancient cave paintings. There is a powerful cultural tradition of the artist as the painter. The figure of painters as artists who can be who they are, who are free, is rooted deep in our cultural traditions. Being an artist explains eccentric behavior; it allows you creative freedom. For people who are ill, seeing themselves as painters frees them to be themselves.

The visual image is a compelling link to guided imagery. When most people think of imagery, they think of visual imagery. The term *visualization,* which is still used for guided imagery, refers to visual images because they are the most accessible images to start with for most people. Visual images transport you to another place. Looking at a painting is no longer habitual seeing; it is something from within you brought to life. When we close our eyes and imagine a scene, we see inward. We are in a place that we can look around in, feel, and move in. It is really a total experience, but the visual modality is the one that most of us are most aware of. It is not visual imagery like the outer world, or like a movie. It is softer, more transitory, faster moving, more like a dream. And that is the place from which we make visual art, the place of softly glimpsed images, the place where images come from. When we start to paint or sculpt, we bring an image outward, whether the image is conscious or unconscious. The image becomes real and we can then see it in the outer world.

When you ask visual artists who work with patients how art heals, they all have different answers. One day we went around a circle and asked all the artists how art heals. One artist said art heals by distraction. It gets people's minds off their illness, and then unconscious healing happens. Another said it

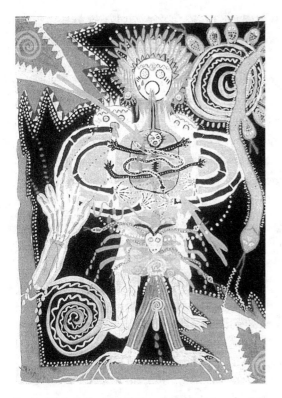

is different for each person—no two people use visual arts to heal in the same way. Another artist said that making healing art is a meditation. A physiological shift occurs when meditation takes place. You concentrate deeply; you go inward. Another artist said that making art is real magic, that a new line on a page where there was nothing before puts the person in the world of creation. Many artists say that making a painting takes you inside. They use the term *elsewhere* and describe it as a feeling of going somewhere else. People call the feeling different things, but everyone knows what it feels like. Another artist said art heals by connecting you to something, to something larger, to your greater self. Most artists-in-residence agree that people can go to a different place with art; people can make art and not be distracted. They can be with themselves differently. They can tap into their healer within. In an objective way, art can help people witness themselves. Art can take a person from the inner world outward to the community. Artists also say that art heals because it is like play; it brings you back to your childhood space.

Denise Bardovi, *Shaman*. Denise created a series of paintings to heal herself of cat-scratch fever and chronic fatigue syndrome. In them, she portrayed her illness, her healing forces and helpers, and her healing. She had not painted until she became ill. Her first paintings were color washes and lines. The series she created is an elegant visual record of the process of how art heals.

Many artists talk about control. Even when you are ill you can still control your art. Art is your own; you have control of all its aspects. You can erase a line, take a whole shape off, change a color. You can manipulate it. You can even tell the artist that you refuse to make art and not do it. Art shifts the person to what psychologists call an internal locus of control. When people become the artists, they have mastery, they lead. A woman recovering from a lung transplant told the artists working with her, "When I make art, I am in control of my body and mind. I have power to reduce fear. I feel my old power come back. Doctors and nurses have told me what to do for months. Now, as a painter, I tell myself what to do. This is the part of my life that is completely mine."

Art is a vehicle to create focused intention. It helps you regain power; it is a tool to concentrate on any aspect of healing you want. This is very different from the medical model. The choice to do art is part of the empowerment. People can make the artist do what they want; they can make anything they want instead of being told what to do.

STARTING OUT: MARY'S STORY OF RECLAIMING HER INNER ARTIST

Both the authors of this book started in healing art as visual artists, Mary as a painter and Michael as a photographer. We will tell you more of Mary's story as a detailed example of someone who healed herself with painting. Her experience happened by itself; she had no one to help her become a healing artist. There was no program in art and healing, and no healing artist nearby. She had never heard of art and healing. It just happened. She had only her friends who were painters to help her start to paint. Her story has many of the aspects we hear from people who start out using visual arts to heal. If she can heal herself with art, you can, too. She was just an ordinary housewife without a healing artist. She did it herself.

> I was always drawn to the visual arts. I loved to look at paintings. When I looked at them, I could go elsewhere. There was a spatial experience in a visionary world, a window into a free state of consciousness. As it engaged my eyes, it engaged my interest and took me inward. So when I became deeply depressed and over-whelmed by my own despair, I knew my medium was paint. There was an agony of despair that ripped my body and I cried for

months. At that point in my life, when I was experiencing such pain, I wondered what I could do to survive. The first time I painted, I got help from a friend who was a painter. Lee Ann took me to her studio the first time and handed me paper and crandache crayons, watercolor crayons, and watercolors. I made my choice of crandache because they were brightly colored, and I liked the way they looked. There were lots of them, in a box like crayons. I had no idea which materials to choose; I just grabbed the ones that appealed to something in me, to my sensuality. Then I started making marks, lines, shapes, and colors. My first drawing turned out to be a still life of the studio. It was clearly what was in front of me that grabbed my eye. It was the lived experience before me. I looked at my life for my point of reference. I did not know what to do, so I just looked around the room. Lee Ann would say, "That was beautiful. What a nice shape. Those colors are great. You are a natural. Oh, Mary, you are an artist." I was confused; I did not know what was happening. The more I painted, the more I was surprised that I could create forms. It was so gestural. Somehow the lines were connected to how I felt. I was surprised by how the medium responded to my emotions better than words. It seemed so preverbal, the medium responding to my sense of creation. It expressed deep feelings that words can't.

Then I looked around and found an image of a distorted woman in a book. I looked at images in my life that resonated with me, that I wanted to look at, that had meaning for me where I was then. I took the woman image as a point of departure. I just took something that I responded to, something that was around me, that came from my experience. I took whatever I recognized, what related to me. I knew somehow I needed to start with images that were immediately available to me, images I could create a dialogue with. I then recreated an image in the painting and needed to relate to the image. I saw the woman in pain. It was how I felt. It was a true rendering of the pain, of the brokenness, almost as if it were talking back to me. I couldn't sort out the images; the painting did that for me. I brought something that was deep inside of me out and released it. There was a huge experience of being released; the image released me from what the image is. I externalized the form. I created a page I could look at and think about. Before, it was inside and could not be seen. The images come from a place before thought. When I allowed them to come through me, they came from before conscious-ness. Then, when they came out, I could make sense of them.

So my process was a shift from the still life that started me out to the picture of the woman. First she looked like a stranger. Then I recognized myself in her. I realized she was me, so I decided to do self-portraits. I got the idea to take pictures of myself in postures that reflected how I felt. I used pictures to render the figures. Then there was another shift. I became totally involved in constructing the forms. When I began to paint myself as the figure, I became absorbed in lines, shapes, the folds of her dress, the fingers receding into the shadows, the lines going into the cloth. Now I was involved not only in the emotions but in the figure in space. This was exciting, because I was using the image to reconstruct my life. I did not know it then, but as I recon-structed the image, I was reconstructing myself. To make the image readable, I remade myself. I went from being bent over, torn, and open to being expanding, to raising my head, to bathing in pure waters. As the images changed in content, my body changed, too. In the space of working things out, the process is unconscious. The process that emerged by itself took me from despair and fear to bathing in water and lying back in my body and looking forward.

The steps of healing yourself as a painter can be seen from Mary's story. First she chose painting because she knew from her whole life that she was attracted to it and that a part of her had always wanted to be a painter. Next she set up a studio and chose which materials appealed to her.

She bravely made the first lines and watched as they turned into something. She saw her illness as her despair and she followed the process to allow it to heal her. She saw the healing take place as she was reconstructed and realized that the art was healing her. During the process, she did not analyze or try to figure it out, she just trusted it and continued to make art. She also felt herself heal and saw herself heal. The steps of choosing a medium, making a studio, choosing materials, making the first line, and watching the healing process emerge and heal you are what we will talk about in this chapter. They are the ways that painting heals. Where does intent come in? Start with intent to heal with art; that is all you need. Trust in the process. Creative healing will do itself. Honor who you are and what you want; hold no value judgments. Let the art heal you.

Where is art coming from? What is the source of desire? All you need is intention to create space, choose materials, make something. All you need to do is to give yourself the space to allow what emerges from you to be seen and to heal. Finally, keep on doing the task; persevere. For the healing artist, creating intention is first. The painting studio is an intentional space where you can release the critic. The goal is to go inside yourself to make art as the doorway to your own health, to your own soul. The path is to go inward in your outer and inner life at once. It is not about approval, about paintings that mean something to someone else. Make healing art with the spirit of befriending yourself. Take pride and joy in your own life. Enter healing by your own generosity of spirit. Make art to help yourself change your life. Honor that you are doing something you need to do to live more fully, to move from one place to another. Healing art is not about material success; it is about you healing from within.

MAKING A STUDIO FOR THE VISUAL ARTS

One of the most important things you can do is start in an accessible way, with a sketchbook. That is a good way to begin drawing. You can choose pencil or pens and a blank book. Take the opportunity to connect to something visually, to draw it. You can take your paints and you can caress the image with your hand. Take the shapes, render forms, become familiar with the way you gesture. You can do this because doing so develops confidence in drawing images and it takes you elsewhere. You take something and look at how the light plays on it, how the wind moves it—you play. Right in the heart of the ordinary day, you take advantage of opportunities that present themselves to see deeply.

Take time among your busy moments to create for yourself an artist's tote bag. Make one that has the materials you want to use and is easy to carry. You can put in watercolors, gouache, a jar with water and a lid, colored pencils, or crandache crayons. It is only important that the materials be accessible to you. You can work anywhere you are comfortable. You can set up in your home, on the kitchen table, go to springs, go out in nature, go by yourself, set up a still life. It is like exercise: you have to do it consistently to enjoy the process. It seduces you into it if it takes up space in your life. The experience will draw you back to it; you will cultivate desires to want to do this.

If you want to set up a studio, a room of your own, a space of your own, spend time in your process. You are making a place to spend time with yourself. You can do this on a lunch hour, or whenever you are free for a while. It is also helpful to seek out relationships with artists or other people who are painting. Get in community. People are sources of inspiration in making art. Watch people painting alongside you. This is a reminder and a refuge. You can share a studio, rent a studio with another artist, or rent a studio in a group space where other artists rent, too.

You can also cultivate a friendship with an artist. In that way you can enjoy a relationship and the artist can become a support person in your process. Talk to them as you go on. This is not therapy; it is community. Be with yourself. Be your own healer, your own therapist. You share with yourself. What is critical is that you are giving yourself time to be with yourself. Take the one hundred dollars you would give to a therapist and make an appointment with yourself to paint. When I started to paint, I did not have a healing artist; I only had a friend who was a painter. She encouraged me to paint, and the healing came by itself. That is why I think it is most important to be with artists. A healing artist is not necessary in this process. It is most important for you to paint, to be with people who facilitate your creativity.

The environment, time, and space are what help you make art. Be in a community that will empower you as an artist.

For sculpture, the studio is similar, but it needs the tools you will use for whatever type of sculpture you are making. The most basic sculpture studio has materials from nature, like feathers, bones, sticks, wood, rocks, and other objects. Beyond that, all you will need is glue, a saw, a hammer, a tape measure, a chisel, sanders, and nails or screws. A workshop can be in a basement, a storeroom, a garage, or a corner of the living room. One ninety-year-old man with prostate cancer made a studio in the corner of his room in an old-age home so he could sculpt. He cut the wood in the basement and brought it up to his room to glue and paint. He made life-size sculptures of beautiful women goddesses that were inspiring to everyone around him and deeply healing for himself.

If you are a photographer, all you need is a camera. The type does not matter. Polaroid cameras, point-and-shoot cameras, and expensive cameras will all work. Each has strengths and weaknesses in the process. A Polaroid camera gives you instant gratification. Many hospital artists use it with patients right in their rooms. You can color the prints, mount them, put them in collages, or hang them as they are. You can put them in a journal with stories or hang them in spirals on the wall. A point-and-shoot takes pictures of excellent quality, has the advantage of portability, and is inexpensive. The prints can be worked with easily since they are not mounted like Polaroids. A complicated camera takes a variety of lenses and is more flexible in exposure and composition. You can have the film developed professionally or do it yourself, and you can use either color or black-and-white film. With color film, you can shoot slides or prints. The darkroom and other elaborate photo materials are optional. You can make a darkroom in an extra bedroom, a laundry room, or a large closet. You can carry water from a bathroom sink. You can block off the windows with cardboard and soft cloth on the edges to keep out the light. All you really need is an enlarger, an easel, a timer, trays, a safelight, a tank, a thermometer, and chemicals. You can even print color yourself or use digital photography with computers.

For crafts, you need to fit your studio to the craft you are working—clay, glass, jewelry, metal, and fiber are all healing. Weaving and quilt making are also deeply healing and have been since women started to make art. Currently, some of the most famous quilt makers and weavers are men. To find out how to make a studio, go to an artist in that medium that you know or take a beginners' course anywhere. Again, your intent is to heal, not to make museum art, so do not worry about being perfect. Just get started. The fascination with your art-making process and your materials will take over and drive you to learn more. The concentration and interest will take your mind off your illness, and you will be transported to a different world. The studio is the place where that world lives. Your vehicle may be a pad and paints or a point-and-shoot camera, but when you pick it up you are a healing artist in your own nonordinary world.

HOW TO HEAL YOURSELF WITH VISUAL ARTS

STEP ONE: STARTING ON THE PATH
- Give yourself time alone to let your healing images emerge.
- Start with a sketchbook, pencils and pens, or a camera.
- Get a journal for writing and drawing every day.
- Make an artist's tote bag with materials that is easy to carry.
- Buy paints or materials that look like they would be fun to use.
- Set up a routine to make art every day.
- Say a prayer for your divine creativity to flow through you.

STEP TWO: THE JOURNEY
- Make an intention to heal yourself with visual arts.
- Release your inner critic; let go of judgment.
- Keep your appointment with yourself to paint.
- Collect more materials that would be fun.
- Make marks or color blotches and play.
- Set objects that you love around your studio.
- Find an artist to become a support person.
- Feel Her love surrounding you.

STEP THREE: DEEPENING

+ Make art every day.
+ Pay attention to your images of darkness and light.
+ Let your healing images emerge.
+ Respond to the materials that capture your attention.
+ Cultivate a vision of looking at the world.
+ Use a camera to create a visual diary.
+ Allow yourself to be connected to Her world of images.

STEP FOUR: TRANSCENDENCE

+ Feel God's power coming through your art.
+ Be compassionate with yourself.
+ Realize that there are no mistakes, only opportunities.
+ Experiment with different materials, shapes, and colors.
+ Listen to music while you work to relax.
+ Art is a meditation.
+ Look for images of light and beauty.
+ Realize that Her vision is your vision.

SACRED TIME AND THE VISUAL ARTS

When you approach the canvas, each minute is full. This is different from rushing to work or driving a carpool. When you make art, time vanishes. If we suspend our distractions, we can go into a moment where we are deeply connected to the place our visions come from, from the past, the present, and the future. You open the doorway for your creativity to come in. If you are totally present, you are in a moment that is connected to all of time. Images deep in your spiritual consciousness emerge in a way that resonates with other people. Somehow inside of yourself is a place like dreams, a void inside of time where images begin. The slowing down of time occurs in between your conscious moments. Seize the moments and experience them fully. Go into a moment and stretch it out. Within a sacred moment, go to the point where you are present in your breathing. In that moment is a moment that is so open it is illuminated. All energy, all images, are there before you know it, before you speak, in the dream space within. That is the place where you begin your healing.

LETTING YOUR HEALING IMAGES EMERGE

When you paint, you start from the spiral of lived experience; you go to the place in your life where you are living what needs to be healed. You go to the physical experience of illness, despair, anger, rage. When you approach the process, you start from a place of pain or fear and paint it. The material you work with is the experience. You paint figures that reflect your own emotions. You use the painting as a way to paint yourself, your lived experience, your world. That is your subject matter; the subject is your life, even if the image is symbolic.

When Mary saw the figure of herself facing forward instead of hiding, she was healed; she then didn't need to paint any more self-portraits. She could then paint other things. When you paint your healing experience, you realize it. You realize how afraid and broken you are. A painting stands still for a moment. You capture something you can be with, a space you can go into, a place to share. A painting is honest. You look at yourself and see what you need and then you give it to yourself. You see the need to take care of yourself, you see yourself love yourself, you see your pain and see that you need to be loved. It is an act of love that you give yourself. It is an act of self-love, but as you paint, you move past self-love to give to others. You cultivate a vision of looking at the world that is deep, that is given to others. The paintings are offerings of an authentic vision of yourself to the world. You almost cannot speak; it is deeper than words. The painting captures an experience that allows others to be there, to look at themselves. You share a way of seeing; you give of yourself as an artist and that becomes your gift.

You are really healed when you love yourself perfectly. Then you can perfectly love the world. Then the only thing you can do is to give your art to the world for the sake of love. Sharing your art is your act of love; that is how you heal yourself and others and the world. This view of art is totally different from the view of galleries that sell art to collectors. It is about healing. Your art is a way to access yourself.

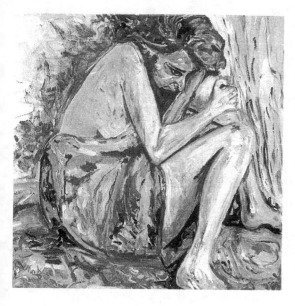

LEFT: Mary Rockwood Lane, *Fear*.
BELOW: Mary Rockwood Lane, *A Stronger Me*.
When Mary painted herself facing forward rather than hiding, she could see that she was healed. These two paintings illustrate how we can see ourselves change before our eyes, in our art.

If you look at the process in slow motion, characteristics emerge. The process is about watching the images appear and letting them grow naturally. It is about honoring what emerges and being open to change. The most powerful images are those that come from deep inside you, that are meaningful to you, that are part of your story or myth. The process is about you taking on your life, trusting your images, trusting them for your art. If you can't think of anything, go with what you see. Take a place in the image you paint and let it go forward to the next one. Then the series grows.

Archetypal images often emerge as you make healing art. In visual portraiture, metaphor emerges. In figura-

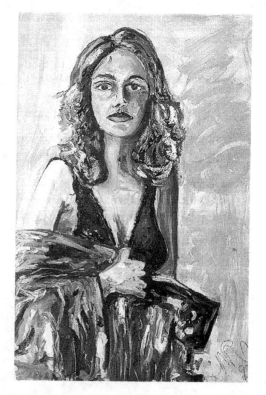

tive painting, symbols appear in the landscapes and still lifes and in the figures you paint. People respond to what they can see. Figures bring you in contact with humanness. They show you yourself and the others around you. They show you family members, relationships, your placement in your environment. You always want resonance, but there are many different types of images that resonate with your life as you live it now. Symbols often appear in healing art unconsciously. Birds, stars, rainbows, houses, hands, trees, and hearts are typical of healing art. The image's content is not important in itself. It is meaningful to the person who paints it. What is more important than the image is the emotional experience of the image. The gesture of the line and the emotional contents are more significant than having the painting look like the person. Rendering accurately is not the point; rendering imagery that is meaningful is what is important.

Surrealist artists portrayed moving into creative space and time as popping through the membrane. They described their experience as going into the body of their lover, going through his or her body, seeing it as transparent, and then moving inside. Many healing artists say that the most significant thing they do is go through a membrane, go elsewhere to a place of beauty inside themselves. They say that only then does She sing to them of the birth of time and space. By Her beauty, they are drawn into Her and through Her, and then they hear Her voice. This journey is portrayed as three drops, each deeper and deeper. The first is leaving ordinary experience, the second is finding the energy of the physical manifestation of forms, and, finally, the third is something coming out of nothingness effortlessly. This process sounds abstract and difficult, but it takes place by itself when you go elsewhere.

When Mary paints, she takes something from her lived experience that is interesting. She says,

> What comes out emerges without thought; what I hope comes out is a gestural movement that I can't conceptualize. I allow the unseen to become seen. You get filled, merge; the seed is born. It is like giving birth. Your body takes control; you don't do anything. In the kitchen, your child brings you a flower. You see it is beautiful, and you want to paint it. Making a painting is like making a salad. It

is really ordinary on the surface. But in painting, you see the ordinary way of being as the greatest joy. You magnify the light in the simple to illuminate the sacred in a new way of seeing. The ordinary mother exists within the extraordinary artist. They exist at once. You look at the flower; you stop time, you create time and space, you are with it and present, beautiful, peaceful, and healing. You go into something visually. The spiral is a soft drop into the place where images come to you like your breath.

Another way of working is to meditate and see the vision and then render it as art. Visionary artists like painter Alex Grey often work in this way. James Surls, a Texas wood sculptor who inspired Michael to conceive his first vision of art and healing, worked with images by seeing them in a relaxed visionary state. He would manipulate the image—rotate it and look at it—in inner space. And then he would bring it out from his personal space of imagery to make art.

Both ways of seeing involve an abstract absorption of power. It is not important which way you use. For Mary, making healing art is closer to making a salad than to intentionally creating a meditative visionary experience. For James, it is an intentional meditative visionary experience. For you, it can be either, totally ordinary or consciously visionary. You start now with the simplest act and move forward. The most important thing is to hold your space, maintaining your relationship to creation.

PATIENT STORIES

Patient stories are our guide to understanding how art heals with personal and powerful imagery. Each of these stories is about making memories and paying attention. The artists who started out in an ordinary experience of just making art found self-love and became enchanted.

Giving Birth to the Earth

When Michael works with cancer patients he is always amazed by the art they bring to their sessions. A woman with bone cancer who had been experiencing only pain and depression started to draw. She brought in drawings of herself that changed from week to week. All Michael did was honor them and help her to look at them with love. If he knew about a symbol, he might tell a story, but he did not interpret her art. At first she drew herself as separated from everything; she was alone, in a box. The drawings were crude, ugly, jarring. She was always trapped, always curled up in darkness. But even then, she loved her drawings. They were surprisingly ugly to her, but she felt right at home in the imagery she drew.

As she drew more, she took the walls away and she became more beautiful. At this point in the process, she became intensely interested in her drawing and spent more and more time doing it at home between sessions for pure enjoyment. The drawing became a preoccupation; it became the most important thing for her to do. As she drew, she almost became wild. She was so full of energy, she could hardly sleep. She woke up and started drawing immediately and sometimes drew late into the night.

Suddenly the drawings changed. The imagery started to be surprising and wonderful. She drew herself flying in space with crystals, with animals. She saw herself surrounded by rainbowlike colors swirling around her, painting her. She saw herself merging with things, blending into light. Finally, the drawings portrayed her giving birth to the earth, an image of union and connectedness that showed who she had become. The drawings were now in astonishing colors; they were shaded and three-dimensional, and they even became illuminated with gold ink. They were graphic representations of the transformation that was occurring. They showed her as healing even before she knew what was happening. They took her animals, her friends, her cat, and, most important, the earth itself and made them all hers. She was now connected to them, part of them, one with them.

Out of Her Cocoon

Both as a patient and an artist, a young woman used her creative resources and empowered herself to become deeply involved in her own recovery from chronic pain. Diagnosed with fibromyalgia, a chronically painful condition that had severely disabled her to the point that she became wheelchair-bound and severely depressed, she began a series of seventy-two drawings that she refers to as *The Journey*. The first painting was called simply *Pain*. After she became engaged in the drawing process, the colors, patterns, and symbols took on significance for her, and her drawings began to guide her in new directions.

She had become extremely sick. She had dropped to ninety-eight pounds and could not work, and she thought that she was dying. She could not communicate with her doctors or nurses and was extremely depressed. She started meticulously drawing her images. She began to draw the pain. She could not communicate it verbally to the staff. They did not seem to understand her constant complaints. She would draw her pain purple and yellow, with spiked balls. She would show electric-current jolts going through her. Her art made her intimate with her pain and her sensations. She drew herself in a cocoon where she was wrapped in pain. Then she began to do landscapes. She became a tiny woman in the landscape in the cocoon, so tiny you could not see her well.

She began to develop a visual way to deal with her pain, to deal with the hospital. Purple and orange colors represented her experience of pain, heart flowers in the landscapes represented self-love, and a frequently recurring drawing of a path represented her journey. She began to see people, to talk about the pictures rather than about her pain. She did this for several months. She would paint little flowers in wild pink colors and then they would grow. Then she had insights of what they meant to her. She did this on her own. She talked about her images but did this on her own. She realized that she had to love herself. She realized this from her flowers. The flowers were self-love. It was like something was talking to her, the images were telling her stories. She saw them evolving over time. Then her intent was to make images to help her in the healing process.

One day she burst out of her cocoon; the butterfly was free. She was then an actively involved artist. She had become more deliberate, not just intuitive. She was now more empowered. She could actually do this, and she drew herself well. From then on, the paintings were a monitor of her pain, and she was outside it enough to be able to express it.

For her, the visual world had become a potent and direct form of communication. She says about the process, "My realization was that if I really wanted to help myself with the pain, I would have to change my whole life. It was in my drawings that I began my search for the person I was born to be." Her drawings reflected her experiences, her relationship with her caregivers, and her relationship with her pain. She shares her drawings with her caregivers as a vital part of her therapy and healing process. When they can see her pain, they believe it and can treat it better. When they see her images of healing, they know medications are effective. Finally, she has become involved with sharing her experience of art in her own recovery process.

"I Take Pictures So I Can Never Forget"

A series of pieces by a woman photographer documents her friend's experience of breast cancer and its treatment. The photographs confront with creativity the experience of a woman living with this disease. The patient shared her response to this documentation: "I want to be able to remember what has happened to me in the last few months. Unlike some women I have read about who don't want to remember, I can never forget. The photographs and my journal will always be a link for me. The words provide an immediate and urgent release for what I'm feeling, and the images document what I'm experiencing." She explains that while exploring the uncharted territory both of having breast cancer and of documenting her healing journey, she feels she is coming out of the closet of social taboo and fear. She shares her humanity and her personal experience boldly. This is a powerful visual narrative through her friend, who has photographed her throughout her treatment.

Mary Lisa Tells How She Started as an Artist-in-Residence

My friend who was a nurse called me to please come down to the hospital. So I brought T-shirts with me and some paints and things. She said, "We have a little girl here who has been waiting to see you. I told her you were coming." She was seven years old. I had never been on a bone marrow transplant unit. I looked through the window and she was so excited. This little girl was all tied up to her intravenous lines. She was jumping up and down— straight up and down—that I was there, and clapping her hands when I walked in. The nurse told me that she had been standing at the window and looking out and waiting for me to come all day. And she was just like, "Are you gonna play with me, are you gonna do this with me, are you gonna—can we paint?" And she was the cutest little girl. I created all these little characters for her, like little friends. I drew little animals that she had in mind. When she said, "Draw my kitty," I would do the kitty and I would put her pajamas on the kitty that I drew for her. Then she'd paint herself as a kitty with her little bunny slippers on and with her little hair barrettes and with her little hats on. She would giggle and draw poodles with little dresses on. This child, who had spent a long time here, at one point would not speak with anybody. She had totally shut down. The only way she would communicate was by making animal noises and drawing with me. They would call me and say, "Can you please come and work with her because she won't talk." Until I got there, she was having a horrible time with the bone marrow transplant. She would be vomiting and then I would come and she would paint and she wouldn't want me to go, you know. There's such tremendous loneliness.

As soon as I walked into the room I knew that this was where I belonged. It was a knowledge that what I do, the person that I am, could provide a service that would be important here. I knew that it was very important work. It was joy. I didn't get intimidated until I got home, because then I'd think about it. It really upsets you because of the love you develop there for the families and the pain that they go through. But I knew that I could do this job. I knew that what I had to offer was very important in this situation. I feel like I'm life. I think I have a sense of their abandonment and I want to listen to them. I want to hear what their story is and I want to make them feel better if I can.

Mary Lisa's Advice on How to Heal Yourself with Visual Arts
The first thing I do when people tell me they can't draw a straight line is tell them, "Excellent, now I don't have to tell you not to do

that." Then, one of the other things I like to do with them is to throw a brush filled with paint onto the paper. I like to work with watercolors. I think watercolors are very easy for people to start out with. Watercolors are water-soluble paints. I use the ones in a tray, any brand will do. With the watercolors, I sometimes have them get a lot of paint on their brush, and then I have them throw the brush at the paper. I have them throw it far if they are resistant. It depends on how resistant they are. They say, "I can't do that, I can't do that" and then I get paint all over the place and they don't care about not being able to do it anymore.

Just the fact that people have to have perfection, that they have the sense that they need to have a photographic image completed or it's not considered artwork, is something I deal with. I start showing them things right away. I'll start showing them that flowers are very simple. If we make a series of circles, then we have created a flower. Now we add a stem. If we roll our brush with the pigment on it, maybe we put another color on the other tip of it and we roll it, we start creating flowers. I'll teach them how to do scribbles with a crayon and then put watercolor washes on there. This is good for all ages. We do scribbling with the crayons and I tell kids they can send someone secret messages this way. They can paint on it and then they can write with white crayons. I have the adults paint a watercolor border around their letters. Maybe they're writing poetry or maybe they're writing notes to their friends. They can draw all these little things in white and then put washes and rainbows of color around it. Another way is to use T-shirts. T-shirts are very nonintimidating, and so I offer my services as someone who will draw for them and then usually their focus is right there on painting that T-shirt. I can get men to paint T-shirts for their children, their grandchildren, their wives, their girlfriends. They'll paint them for somebody. I can get teenage boys to paint T-shirts for their girlfriends.

A T-shirt seems very ordinary, not too emotional or spiritual, but I'll tell you a story. One day I came into the unit and a man came up to me and said, "You are the one." I immediately thought, "What have I done?" I felt guilty. He told me that I had changed his life and he thanked me and hugged me. I had worked with his wife, who was very ill. She wanted to paint a T-shirt for her young son. She knew her little boy loved vacuum cleaners, so she started to paint a vacuum cleaner. I helped her. As she worked, she became more and more absorbed in the process. As she painted, she could hear her son running up and down in the hall outside her room making the sounds of a vacuum cleaner and it would make her smile and cry at once. And she became sicker and sicker. She concentrated as hard as she could on the colors, the shapes, the background. And one day I came to work and I heard she had died. The next day, her husband showed me what he had done. He had framed the T-shirt so lovingly and beautifully. He told me it was the last thing she had done for her little boy. It was her last gift to him and they would treasure it always. It was her love to him expressed as art. It was only a T-shirt, only a vacuum cleaner, but it was as deep as this work gets.

In general, when painting on paper, start with watercolors or acrylics because they're both water based. Use pencils, crayons, and watercolor pencils because you can re-mark them and add wash and experiment with them with a little more control. You can shape the paper into a circle or other shape; you can make a mandala. Sometimes just changing the shape of the area and adding colors will help. Experiment with paper wet or dry, lots of paint, a little paint, a little dot, a big dot; experiment with where the colors fall and how they blend together and just be fascinated with what happens. Later on, you can start putting things in, really focusing more and tuning in to your feelings. Just allow yourself the opportunity to play with that a little and get to know your medium. Let yourself go and ask, "What could happen here?" And then you'd be surprised at how quickly your accidents and things you fell into—things you had no intention of displaying—become art. You get impressions from the way your colors have shown up on the page. The story you create inside yourself is very important; it's your story.

Lee Ann Tells about Starting Out as an Artist-in-Residence

Lee Ann Stacpoole is a multitalented artist whose medium changes with the changes in her life. Lee Ann was the very first artist-in-residence at Shands Hospital, University of Florida, Gainesville, who conquered her fear of going into an environment she was unsure of. She was the first to work with people who were not artists. She taught us that everyone is an artist. With her soft encouragement and empowerment she allowed each person to find his or her own area of creativity. When you would paint with her, she would say, "That is the most beautiful painting I have ever seen." And you would say, "Really?" and she would say, "Yes, I wish I could paint like that. Look at the way you make this mark." Instead of you saying, "I wish I could paint like you," she said it first. As she sat next to you with her long blond hair, her dress that flowed like silk of a bright wild green that shimmered like light, her Native American earrings and necklace, she made you feel like an artist. Her arms were always soft and gentle. In her voice you could sense that she knew you could make art. She would tell you that she was a self-taught artist and that she believed if she could do it, you could do it, too. Lee Ann was also the artist who set up the project to have children with cancer and their families paint tiles to go up on a tile wall. Her son Daniel was born with Downs syndrome, and she is working on a photography project to sensitize people to see developmentally handicapped children as beautiful.

Lee Ann Stacpoole tells this story about seeing the first patient, Michelle, in the Arts In Medicine program.

> When we started in AIM we bought tons of art supplies. We bought crandache paints, black hardback journals, water paints, Fimo clay. Everything was beautiful, brightly colored, and rich. We walked into a patient's room and we were starting out on a journey so beautiful we could not imagine where it would lead. The first patient was fourteen years old. She was bald from chemotherapy. She had a bone sarcoma. She had been an artist in school; it just seemed like a wonderful opening. And as we walked into the room, we said to ourselves, "We will be an artist and make art," and she was sweet and receptive. We gave

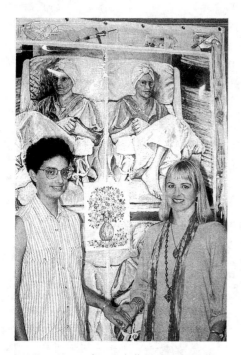

Lee Ann Stacpoole, *Michelle's Flowers*. Making art creates long-lasting relationships. Michelle and Lee Ann became friends as they made art together. Michelle's painting of flowers takes the center place among the portraits Lee Ann painted of Michelle as she was getting chemotherapy on the bone marrow transplant unit. Michelle's painting was made with the mouth swabs she used for her painful mouth care. This painting of the portraits and the flowers was exhibited in a local gallery and became a most compelling example for the community of how art and healing are one. It enabled people to see more deeply into Michelle's experience as she allowed herself to be seen. And we thank her for that.

her materials to paint with and the next day we saw that the art box we had left for her was right where we put it.

Imagine it was you going into the room. Picture yourself as the artist-in-residence, just starting out in unknown territory. Maybe poetry would work, you think as you seek for forms. And as the patient sits in a chair in the tiny dark room with the curtains drawn around her, it seems somber and quiet, and she looks at you with eyes so old they seem ancient. She is always in different moods; she is consumed by sadness, by anger, by frustration— like many teenagers but more so, here in this dark place. But she doesn't engage you at all. Although you are with her, you are confused. Then you realize you cannot make her draw, you cannot make her write. You deal with who you are as a person, with your big ideas and passion. You sit on the bed with her, you start to talk to her mother, you do the best you can.

Then you realize that the only thing you can do is draw her. You draw her in all her changed moods.

You see her as so beautiful. Now she is open. As you spend time with her, you realize that painting her brings you two together.

With these prolonged encounters, where you sit and draw, there is room for conversation to come out of nothingness. Your agenda is dropped; you are doing what you are doing as an artist. You are doing what you know how to do. You bring beauty into the dark, compressed space, where before there has only been sickness. You have a relationship with her now that is significant, and the relationship you have is deep and intense. You have seen her; she has seen you. It is different from every other relationship you have ever had. You want nothing other than to help her.

And then Michelle goes home. You get a letter from her mother that she is going back to school. You get a letter from Michelle herself. Inside the letter is a small painting made with the cotton swabs she used when she had the mouth sores. She had to use these swabs three times a day during the most painful part of the bone marrow transplant to care for her mouth, which was eroding with the chemotherapy. You knew the mouth swabs were the most painful part of her hospital stay. And she painted a bouquet of flowers with these swabs for you. She painted this for you to have. It was like an incredible gift. You don't know what effect you had, but you realize it was monumental. It was so meaningful to her as her artist that she turned her pain into flowers for you.

And you take her little painting and position it in the center of the portraits you had made as her moods changed, and you see her as beautiful, and you create a piece called *Michelle's Flowers*. The piece takes form and is a monument to this first experience of art and healing. It is about simply being with her. It is about having no expectations and simply having the intention to heal. It is about art as a way of caring, a way of reaching out and being connected to somebody in a more meaningful way than we have the opportunity to be in our ordinary lives. It is an experience where you get goose bumps and are actually touched as you touch someone else.

Lee Ann's Advice

Keeping a journal and painting on a piece of paper or cutting out pictures and pasting them on is a good way to begin. Listening to tapes of music while you paint works well to relax you. There are lots of different materials, and maybe one material isn't the right way for you, so try different media. I like gouache better than watercolors. They're both water-based mediums, but gouache has more of a gutsiness to it, a richness and saturation to the color. You can go from light to dark and dark to light with gouache. With watercolors, you can only work from light to dark. I think gouache is much more forgiving and easier for people. I like the water-soluble sticks and pencils that they can draw with. Just make drawing marks either with a stick or with a pointed pencil and then use a water brush to soften it or make it all kind of blur. I always encourage people to use the best kind of materials they can afford to get. But other than that, use anything, typewriter paper, even the back of a grocery sack.

There is no right or wrong; there is no bad art. Everything, every mark that you make, is a potential part of a creative process that I believe helps you, helps your inner self. It's a freeing; it's opening a door for you. Just go ahead and make that mark, and give yourself permission to make the next one. The more you do it, the more easily it will flow. When you say, "I never can learn how to draw," I say, "Can you write the ABCS?" and you say, "Yeah, of course," and I say, "Well then you can learn to draw. It just takes time." You have to learn how to see what you're looking at.

Try to find out what in your past had caused limitations. Usually when people tell me that they want to be an artist, something had stopped them at some point from doing it. I'd say, "Play with your materials. Just explore." Do you want to paint flowers? Landscapes? Do you want to paint designs? Pick something out of a magazine, a little something that you like, and try to look at it. Do it, do it, and do it, again and again. In doing it, you will get better. The more you do it, the better you will feel about your work. Do not worry about criticism. This is about healing, not perfection.

Well, the first major experience I had with healing art was working with Mary. Mary came to me and was so interested and she wanted to watch me draw and to watch me in my process. It wasn't that I minded her watching, and I was glad to have her there, but I really sensed that she needed to be making art. She said, "Oh, but I can't do it. I've tried, I've taken classes. I just can't do it." And I said, "Well, what kind of classes have you taken?" And I found out she had taken classes from a woman who does very detailed, beautiful watercolor paintings. Well, here was Mary. Anyone who knows Mary for five minutes knows she is not the kind of person who is going to sit there with a tiny little brush and do these delicate little watercolor paintings. She just was using the wrong medium. So I gave her these sticks, kind of like oil pastel or, actually, water-soluble color sticks—they don't have points or anything—and I said, "Just go for it. Just start playing." I said, "Just do it," and I was blown away. Not only did she just do it, but she did it like it was a high-speed train going by the studio. I was really blown away. I thought, "This woman has so much art in her. She is just bottled up." I think it was like a genie trying to get out of a bottle where there's only a pinhole and he can't squeeze through. Mary needed a little bit more space. Mary always was an artist; she just needed to know that for herself. She needed to give herself the permission and recognition that her inner self was beautiful. She needed to know that what she made with her inner self in that process was wonderful and that there was no right or wrong attached to it. It was what it was and it was radiant. That was my first experience.

I knew that it would be good for her. There was one day I made her cry because I kept saying, "Say 'I am an artist'" and she said, "I can't, I can't." I've been through therapy, and it wasn't that we were doing therapy with each other. But I did see Mary get better, healed. We didn't use the word *healed*, but we thought it.

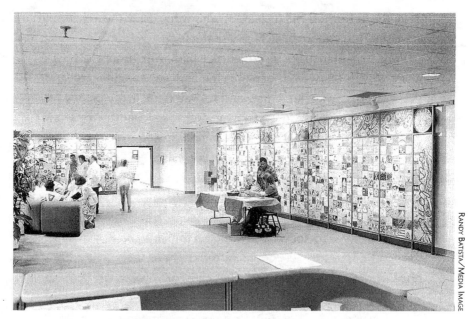

Lee Ann Stacpoole, *The Tile Wall, Shands Hospital.*
The healing tile wall is the illumination of embodied moments of making art. In a studio adjacent to the radiation oncology center, the child with cancer, the parents, and the staff could come in and paint a tile. Each tile told a story. The tiles were hung in the tile wall of over one thousand tiles that now hangs in the hospital atrium for people to see each time they come to the hospital.

There are no mistakes, only opportunities to explore the infinite possibilities of painting.

Lee Ann Tells Stories about the Tile Wall

I created a project that allowed children with cancer, their families, and the medical staff who took care of them to paint ceramic tiles. They worked together in a studio set up in the waiting room of the cancer center. One day this family came in, a large extended family. It seems like six or seven people came into the studio together. The child who was ill in the family had on a mask; it was hard for him to hold a brush or a pencil because his hand was shaking so much from weakness. I watched the father take his son's hand, place it on the tile, and draw the outline around his son's fingers. He then helped his son in starting to paint his hand on the tile. The child painted the dark brown color of his skin with his father's help. The father was also painting his own tile. I remember watching this father hold his son's hand and observe his son's fingernails so that he could draw fingernails on the hands on the tile. It was such a beautiful act of love that I was privileged to see that day. This whole family surrounded this boy with love, and you really felt that this love and what they were going through transcended his illness; that seemed real clear from all the tiles each member of that family did. It was a beautiful moment to watch and to see. In normal everyday life, lots of parents never have the chance or the time to sit down with their children and do something like painting together or doing a project together. What was really nice about the tile project was that it gave the families a few moments to do that together in the midst of all their scheduled doctor's appointments and treatments. This took them away for a while. I really think that's what I saw that year with most of the people who walked through the door.

We began, at a certain point, to ask the participants if they were willing to answer a couple of questions. One was, "What does your tile mean to you?" And the second one was, "Did you feel any different while you were painting your tile?" We asked that second question because of one woman. This woman came in and she was happily painting this wonderful picture of a happy lady with an Egyptian hairdo and these wild earrings, and she was just the most bubbly woman in the world. We asked her if she was sick and she said, "Oh yes, I've had so much pain—I've just had this really, really horrible pain with this illness and it's just been the worst thing." We were sitting there looking at her and she didn't look like she was in pain at all at that moment, and I said, "I hope you don't mind my asking, but do you notice when you are painting that maybe you feel a little better?" She looked startled and she thought to herself and she said, "Well, you know, I didn't notice my pain. I did feel better while I was painting." While she was verbalizing about all her terrible pain, she was happily painting away on her tile as if she was out on a picnic!

When I did the tile wall, I gave people some very basic, simple steps. We would show them how to use the materials. We would explain to them that the colors would change somewhat when they were fired, although most of them stayed the same. A blue would be a blue and what you saw as green would be green. Some changed radically, but we had a sample tile showing the fired colors. They could choose which colors they wanted to use; they could choose what kind of brush they wanted to use, whether a big one or a little one. We told them that they could draw their image first with a pencil or pen and that anything they drew would burn off in the firing process, so there was no way to make mistakes. We had to constantly tell people, "It's okay, this isn't a mistake." One of the things I did frequently to help people loosen up was to say, "See, you can have fun going like this," and I'd paint a little swirl and dab on little blobs. I'd say, "Dr. Graham-Pole, the pediatric oncologist physician who cofounded the Arts In Medicine program, comes in here and puts all these little blobs of color on the tile and they're really pretty when they're fired." They'd see one of his tiles and figure that if a doctor could play with color, they could, too. I'm sure they were saying this to themselves and feeling better.

Cecelia on Breast Cancer and Transcendence

Cecelia Thorner is a breast cancer survivor who makes sculpture warrior shields. Before she started making her fabric art, she was a mother and had run a clothing business. She had never made art or been an artist. Since she has had breast cancer, her life has changed. She is now an artist. She has made a series of shields over many years that are powerful and transformative to her and to others who see them. She is a wonderful example of a person who started as an ordinary woman and became an artist healer. She made art to heal herself and through the process became a powerful woman and an artist.

When you see Cecelia you are struck by both her beauty and her sense of self. She holds her head high like a warrior and her eyes look directly at you. She looks at everything around her with intensity, she is so alive. Her shields take your breath away. Women with breast cancer look at her shields and their hair stands on end.

> I have to say that I didn't plan what the pieces were; they just came from my unconscious. There were times when I would try to manipulate what I was going to do. It did not feel right and I couldn't allow myself to do it. I discovered that if I just let go and let my unconscious mind—the spiritual part of me—come out, these wonderful pieces were created. I wasn't quite sure with each one what they really were about as I made them, but by the time I finished the piece, it really became clear what it was, what aspect of myself it represented. I spent a lot of time walking by myself. Not going on a walk with the intention of coming up with answers, but just going on a walk and kind of freeing my mind of clutter. It was amazing that these revelations would just come up, and I would write them down. I kept a journal, but it was very informal.

> At the end of three years I had made eleven pieces, and after I had finished the eleven pieces, another revelation occurred. I saw that in the beginning, all my pieces were very large and my art was kind of looking at the whole philosophical aspect of breast cancer and the parts that were really not very scary. But then, as time went on, at the very end, all my pieces became smaller and smaller. Those were the pieces that were really about the difficult part—that I might die—and all of these very, very scary things. It had been eighteen years and I was just so emotionally drained. But it was at that point that I really felt that I was healed. I had gotten over the trauma and I could just let go of that part that I had dealt with for so long. It was kind of like starting all over again. I mean, I felt really free. The other way of looking at it is that in the beginning, the large pieces represented this huge enormous hole in me and as I began to make the

pieces, the hole kept getting smaller and smaller and smaller until it finally just closed up and healed.

My series was called *Warrior Woman* and it was about becoming a warrior to be able to fight breast cancer. One of the last pieces that I did I called *Warrior Woman—Wings of Transcendence*. It was very winglike, and there was a body and it was very feminine. I had completed the piece and I had sent the slide off to be included in an exhibit for women who had had breast cancer. It was accepted, but I was not happy with the piece—there was something wrong with it—so I completely took it apart. I was really frustrated and I thought that I had really not transcended; it just had not happened. I tried a lot of different things, and a month or so went by, quite a long time, and I went on a walk and I just decided that I was going to let go of it. When it came together, it would be together, and it could be today or it could be next year. So I came home from my walk and I had all the pieces disassembled on my deck and I looked—and the answer was there.

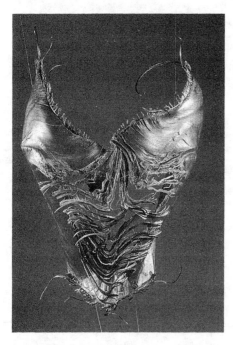

Cecelia Thorner, *Warrior Woman—Wings of Transcendence*. Cecelia had never made art until she made fiber shields to help heal herself from breast cancer. She says, "To me, the piece is about a woman. She's transcending. She's going into a place where she's never been before and it's symbolic of my allowing myself to go within. Inside here is this vibrant, creative, passionate woman that I don't think I ever allowed myself to see. It's very frightening and scary to see her, particularly after breast cancer. Breast cancer takes away from the feelings of passion and creativity."

It was the most awesome experience. I'm not sure that I really believe in God, but that day I felt that there really is something more. I was allowing myself to see that, and I think that was probably one of the most thrilling moments of my life. It was also about trusting myself to listen to what my inner voice was telling me, and maybe not understanding at the moment, but just following my instinct. I just kind of felt like, I'm the vehicle and there is something greater in me. I've tapped into that and I'm making these things that hopefully other people will see and they will be transformed, too.

Well, even now when I speak of that experience, I have to take this deep breath. I grew up as a Methodist and you go to church and you hear all these incredible stories about a Godlike experience. I have to say that, for me, it was the same. The incident was about discovering that there is something greater within your own self. You don't really need to go outside of yourself to be whole.

I think I just felt that if there is a God, that he was telling me that there was a message I was supposed to be getting. I just remember feeling it was the most awesome kind of experience. I think doing these pieces, all of them, has probably been one of the most meaningful things I've ever done in my life.

To me, the piece is about a woman. She's transcending. She's going into a place where she's never been before and it's symbolic of my allowing myself to go within. Inside here is this vibrant, creative, passionate woman that I don't think I ever allowed myself to see. It's very frightening and scary to see her, particularly after breast cancer. Breast cancer takes away from the feelings of passion and creativity.

Another thing occurred with regard to this piece. I finished it, and I knew it was perfect and fabulous, and I put it together in not a very long time, just a few hours. I have a wall set up with the correct lighting and I hung it on the wall and I turned on the light and I looked at it and the inside part of the shield was glowing red—I mean it was like the most frightening, exciting, exhilarating experience. That was absolutely unplanned. It was just wonderful because it truly was alive—it represented life.

Cecelia's Advice on Starting to Heal Yourself with Visual Art

I advise women who have breast cancer, or anyone who wants to heal themselves with art, to start by tapping into the possibilities of what really is within you. I suggest writing, talking into a tape recorder, meditation, making sure that you spend some time alone. Try not having music on, but really being quiet. It doesn't mean sitting in a lotus position meditating—it could be walking, or just sitting. This allows you to hear all of these voices inside you; it allows you to tap into your gut feelings, into your intuition. You start to believe in your intuition, and realize that that really is your true life.

RELEASING YOUR INNER CRITIC

For most people, one of the first things they face is a voice inside of them that says, "You can't do this, you are not good enough, this is silly, you are not an artist." So one of the first major goals is to tell yourself, "It is all right." Release yourself from your inner critic. Don't censor yourself—be free to make art in a state of exhilaration. Have no judgment—tell your self-critic to go into another room and rest awhile. Make art like a child would. Hopefully, as a child your critic was not born yet. You created art for the experience of doing it. You allowed it to happen. Let go of "I can't do it." Think "Yes, I can." This will take you from where you are inhibited to where you are free. When you start to make art, tell yourself you will make art no matter what. Tell yourself that your life depends on this. This is one choice you will make to heal, this is one choice you will make to save your life.

When you get ill or depressed or have a life crisis, you adjust your priorities. When a person gets a diagnosis of cancer or is so depressed they can't go on, everything changes in one moment. The inner critic drops off suddenly and is replaced by "What I have to do is primary. No matter what I think, I need to do this now" and "When I make art with an intention to heal, no one can ever take it away from me." The feedback of success is so powerful it takes over everything. You know you are an artist no matter what anyone thinks. You are full inside; there is no longer room for criticism. It is also important in releasing the inner critic to realize that healing art is not about success, aesthetics, or making art that another person likes. It is about healing. No art you make is bad, or wrong. It is what you are doing to heal yourself, others, or the earth. It is that simple. Repeat this to yourself if your critic pipes up.

Gina Talks about Compassion, Body Feelings, and Healing

Gina Halpern is a ceramics artist and painter who has been using art to heal for twenty-five years. She is one of the most innovative people in this field. She has made mandalas with cancer patients, where she paints what the person sees. She has worked with clay in hospital lobbies, she has danced and made music with children, and she has taught workshops on art and healing at many conferences nationwide. She is the artist who made the mandala with Michael's wife, Nancy, when Nancy had breast cancer. She healed herself of a critical illness with art, and after that experience set up Healing Through Arts, one of the first organizations in art and healing.

Gina often dresses in bright colors, like a figure in one of her paintings. She sometimes dresses like a clown because she has been a clown with children who were ill. She stretches out her hands while she talks, as if she is dancing. Her eyes are bright and she cares deeply for the people she works with.

> I was in my mid-twenties and I had a major illness. I had had a Dalkon Shield and I developed pelvic inflammatory disease and they didn't know what it was. I spent the first months dealing with that in a little hospital in Maine, scared out of my mind. They put me on medication and on my twenty-fifth birthday I had a drug reaction that almost killed me. I think I was a lot closer to death than I realized. I was sick beyond belief. I remember that for my birthday, somebody brought me a large Italian bowl. It was the only visual reference I had in the whole room and so it became the focal point. When I was just afraid and in pain, I would find myself staring into this bowl. I realized later that it was my first experience of a mandala—the use of an image as a focusing device—and that became a really important discovery for me.
>
> Then I began to photograph the objects on the bedside table. I had a close friend bring my camera and I would photograph the shelves and the flowers. I realized that when I was looking through the camera, I was not afraid, I was not in pain. I would go into the beauty of an object and lose myself in it for a small period of

time. That was an extraordinary discovery, and as long as I was involved in the art and the beauty, I was not in the suffering and in the fear. I thought, "What if I could consciously make art with that intention for other people?" The illness became the doorway for me into the spiritual. I got so close to death that I had to start asking some big questions. I knew that for me, the way to understand this whole phenomenon of illness was through art. Art was the only way that I could articulate what I was experiencing, what my fear was, what my longing was, what the spiritual encounters that I was having that I didn't have words for—what they were. I could express that all through the art.

When working to heal others, I would first say, there is a window—you know, there's this place where you leave the ego outside. There is this window of clarity that happens, a presence that happens. When I was studying psychology, we used to talk about the power of presence, a healing presence. When I started studying Buddhism, there was a meditation that I found on the Buddha of Compassion. The meditation starts off with he or she—however you want to look at this deity—gazing at you with compassionate eyes and seeing you completely with love. They see you inside and outside. Just letting yourself be seen compassionately is an enormous thing.

The three main components of working with others for me are attention, intention, and compassion. You have to start with yourself, which is the hardest thing. The first time I tried it, I couldn't sit and be gazed upon with those compassionate eyes. If I was going to teach any doctor, any nurse, this would be the meditation I would start with because it's like the quintessential piece of healing, whether it's healing with medicine or healing with art or healing as a chaplain. In the visualization, you let yourself be seen compassionately by the Buddha, the compassionate one, and then you imagine the Buddha entering your body and filling you up to the very capacity, to the very edges of your skin, and you see the world through the Buddha's eyes. You see through the eyes of compassion. You are yourself, but you're also seeing through the eyes of compassion, so if you are basically a judgmental person, or you have expectations, you need to give yourself over to the one who fills you and gives you the ability to have compassion. When you are present with another person and see that person without judgment but only with love and acceptance, what you see is his or her beauty and uniqueness. When I go to work with someone, that's what happens. I'm still there, but that presence is more there than I am.

This morning when I was working with a man with cancer, I could feel it happening. It has a physiological feeling to me. Things start to hum and I feel a sense of energy that is very palpable. I feel it most when I'm working with others. When I sing—the singing is vibration, right?—when I sing, the goal is to get a kind of resonance. When you sing and you start to resonate, the body feels like it is humming. It's in the front of your nose, but it goes up into your head and it also goes down into the whole chest cavity and the abdomen and everything starts to hum. You're also breathing differently, and that is a very traditional kind of yoga quality. When I get going into this state, it's almost as if the quality of light were shifting.

The light brightens and you know, it's very interesting. I had one vision in which I could see that everything is really energy. What we think of as solid—your body, my body, the table, the chairs—is really just molecules of atoms vibrating at different frequencies and densities, and what we see as the illusion of reality is really just all vibration of energy. The other night I actually dreamed of going to make art on an ice cap, like a polar ice cap, and it was all translucent, but when the light came through it, I saw the fractal crystalline patterns illuminated in turquoise and magenta and I could almost again see the molecular structure vibrating.

This morning I worked with a man who's dealing with metastasized prostate cancer. In this work, I'm a scribe. I set my ego aside and I become the eyes and the hands of the person I'm working for. I make an empty space for the person's visions to come in and fill me and be translated through my talent or gift or whatever you want to call it. It's actually sometimes easier to do it for others than it is to do it for myself. When I was sitting with this man this morning talking, and he was telling me his dreams and visions, everything started to vibrate and I realized it was happening and I had to put my feet on the ground and kind of bring myself back because it's almost, like, too easy to get into an altered state. It's especially necessary to be centered when I'm working with someone else, because the whole goal is to be present for them.

Gina's Advice on Letting Go of Judgment and Making Healing Art

The first thing I would say is that you have to make a space of not judging yourself as an artist or a nonartist. I think that the practice of the Buddha of Compassion is helpful. You can call it Christ or Christ-consciousness, but be with someone who is compassionate. If your grandmother is the most compassionate person you have ever known, imagine that you are sitting across from your grandmother, and she is looking at you with total love and acceptance. Just sit there and be with that person and allow yourself to be seen and ask him or her to help you not be judgmental of yourself as you enter into the process. That, to me, is a really big starting place, because the first thing that stops someone from doing anything creative is "I can't draw, I can't paint, I can't sing, I'm too fat to move" and all the negative judgment. And then you can't go anywhere. But if you feel you can let yourself be seen compassionately, that is a place to begin.

If you can't do the meditation, say or write on the first page of your sketchbook, "I give myself permission to enter this creative experience for my own healing and my own joy and my own peace of mind." Say it—as a beginning statement. That is where I would begin. I might even begin by writing it and coloring around it over and over again with all my favorite colors and just see what happens.

The questions I ask my students are: What is your wound? What is your suffering? What is your joy? What do you need in this minute? What is your healing? And when you think of these questions, create a symbol. I think it is important for people to make the invisible visible. So I think that developing a symbolic language that speaks to you of your experience is very important. Symbols are very powerful, and whether it is a religious icon or a No Smoking sign or a stop sign, it conveys much more than words. So you want to create a symbol for yourself of your healing. Sit and close your eyes and see yourself being seen with love and compassion and nonjudgment. Give yourself permission to make art, to make a symbol. It can be very simple. Picture a blank movie screen behind your eyes, and onto that project a symbol of your illness, or of what you need right now.

For example, I need to be held, so I ask myself, "What do I need?" I might take my hand and put it on the paper and color inside of it with all my favorite colors. When you begin to sit, check in with your body; ask yourself, "What is hurting right now?" Then, as you are drawing, hold the awareness of how you feel now. Or if you disappear into the process of drawing, when you are finished drawing, say, "How do I feel now?" A tool is to take your own pulse, count the number of beats as you count to ten. As you draw, check your pulse and see if there is any change. As you give attention to who you are working with, also give attention to yourself.

When I work with symbols, I ask people to define them as a shape or movement in the air in front of them to get it in their bodies. And they hold that in their bodies. Now that I work with music, I have people write down phrases for the symbol that they can sing. If you are by yourself, practice a chant or a mantra. Experience it with your body and your mind and see how many modalities you can discover.

For materials, I suggest using whatever you are not going to feel intimidated by. Give yourself permission to have an extraordinary experience. So if you are afraid, go for whatever is least scary. It can mean using Xerox paper and a box of crayons, or felt-tip markers from the five-and-ten. I used to tell people to get the big box of sixty-four colors and try them; see what you like, what you hate. Watercolors are very evocative as a material, but they are hard to control. People get frustrated by them. Lots of people love felt-tip markers because the colors are more primary and very direct.

VIEWING ART TO HEAL YOURSELF

It is very beautiful and meaningful to hang the art you make on the walls so you can live with it. You can do this in your studio, your bedroom, your hospital room, or even your kitchen. An important process occurs when you live with your images, as they tell a healing story in time. Sometimes your images don't speak to you as you are making them because they come from a place that is far below where words are formed. Your healing art comes from a place where images are formed, a place that is preverbal. There is no criticism; you have let the forms or shapes begin to emerge without thinking or even making up a story about them. They may exist in the unconscious, in unknowingness.

Then there is an opportunity to allow you to let your images be in your life, to let them tell you stories. As time goes on, you can keep the images as a personal diary. You can hang them around you, put them in a place you can go back to. You can put them away and bring them back out six months or a year later. Then you may see that they tell a story. You can understand yourself in time, sometimes in the future. It is an expressive mode. The healing is the pure mode, the healing is in the release; it is not definable. When you go back and look at it, there is distance, a space. You can tell a story about yesterday better than about the life you are living now. Create space for that kind of dialogue to emerge. When you look at the art you have made, eventually you see who you are. As you look at the images that have emerged, you see what you have been doing, you hear the story of what happened as you healed yourself.

The art that you hang to heal you does not have to be art that you made. You can collect art and buy art that is alive. The art you put up around you can be filled with power or peace. You can choose art you recognize, that speaks to you. When Mary was an art collector, she would find powerful pieces to help her heal. Hanging those paintings that have special significance to you makes your home a healing environment. Whenever you look at the paintings, they reflect where you are. They tell your story. You are able to evoke a personal experience when you look at a painting. Mary describes this: "When I bought a painting of a horse flying over a rainbow, my innate imagery space expanded. I could understand myself better when I bought a painting. When I looked at a painting, I could go between worlds. I could share the images with the artist. I could integrate my life without doing the painting myself. It was about going elsewhere. By going into the painting, there is an opportunity to create new spaces in my world."

You can make a healing art collection for yourself and surround yourself with the images. You can find goddess art and make the goddess live with you. You can find art of animals you love, flowers you love, places you love. You do not need to know why you buy it, but you will know how it affects your life. You can surround yourself with art that embellishes your world. You can populate your world with imagery that is meaningful to your life. Viewing art itself is without distraction. It takes you deeper inside yourself to a place that is meditative and healing.

Going to a museum or to art galleries gives you the opportunity to have an array of experiences. The art can be wild, exuberant, exciting. It depends on what type of imagery you view. If you need energy, you can look at wild paintings. If you need to relax, you can look at soft imagery. A wide variety of art can heal—images of the beach, of animals, of nature, of seeds, of water lilies. Anything that resonates with you in the center of your body, that stimulates your imagination, creates movement, can be healing. Viewing visual art creates healing by moving you, by making shifts, by awakening meaning, deepening understanding, relaxing you, and taking you elsewhere.

SEVEN

HEALING YOURSELF WITH THE WORD: WRITING, POETRY, STORYTELLING, AND THEATER

This chapter offers you the opportunity to invite a writer-in-residence to support you in your inner journey. Like a spirit guide she can help you to make and say words. She always reminds you to be yourself. Allow the spirit of the writer to fly into your life.

INTRODUCING YOUR WRITER-IN-RESIDENCE

Her red hair flows in the wind as she runs. Her cape and scarves float in a spiral. When she comes into the room, her energy is wild; she speaks in a whirlwind of words. Her enthusiasm and energy overflow. She is always the first to share with other artists and staff in clinical artists' rounds at the hospital. She says, "Hi there. I had an exciting week. Listen to my poem, look at my journal with its brightly colored pictures of beautiful songs. I will bring you astonishing life and surprises. I will write you a story you will love; I will put it in a journal for you with wonderful pictures. I am Jan, the writer-in-residence, and I fly in with the wind." And as her books fly open, her pages of pictures show what her patients have been thinking. She makes hand-outs of their printed poems and passes them around like spring flowers.

Jan Swanson was the first writer-in-residence in the Arts In Medicine program at the University of Florida, Gainesville. She established the Accidental Poets Society there and *Zine* magazine, a journal for children in the hospital who had cancer, giving them a place to have their own writing published.

HOW WORDS HEAL

When you write to heal, let the words flow out from within you. Let the words resonate with your spirit. They will bring with them deep memories of words you have heard. It is like letter writing from your heart. Allow the letters to be received. Allow yourself to have the spaciousness so that whatever you write is received as an offering. Words are created from deep within and released into the world. We can shift and change and transfer to a reality that is healing. The words take us deep into our visions or memories, away from worry or pain. They show us new ways of seeing.

When you write, the story emerges in front of your eyes. The beauty of poetry cloaks your life in beauty. The poetry takes you to the essence of what you are looking at. The words are a dialogue reflected back to us. We hear ourselves think. We look at ourselves differently. We create characters that personify aspects of ourselves we do not otherwise face or see, bright and dark sides. We create aspects of ourselves as guides and converse with them. When we tell a story, figures emerge who speak to us from deep within us or from far away. But it is not the voice of our personality. It is the voice of our soul. We have simple instructions that are easy to follow. It is easy to create stories in your life that are like living myths. It is important to create meaning in your own life with your own story. You can bring in your own symbols and discover your own places of magic.

Writing fills the need to be alone, the need to take time to be with yourself. Let the words flow out of you. Don't edit or censor them; let them flow out of your body. Tap into your own soul's most powerful imagery. You translate your own imagery and put it to words. Create a space to write. Place a value on your time to write. It is a lifelong process, so make it easy. You can use a laptop, a computer in a room, a spiral notebook, a journal, anything. You can do it in the evening before going to bed to shed yourself of worries and thoughts of the day. Or you can write early in the morning as you rise to ready yourself for the day. Writing organizes you; it helps you put down thoughts that can change your way of looking at the world. The words can help you make things happen. The writing is a bridge; the first step is seeing and taking action.

From our experience with patients who create healing writing, we can tell you not to be afraid of poetry. Poetry is easy, short, intense. It does not have to rhyme or have any form. It can be like a free-form journal entry. Patients with cancer in the Commonweal Cancer Retreats in Bolinas, California, write poetry on one of the evenings of the five-day retreat, and it is always deeply moving for them and the staff. If you find you like poetry, you can write down lines as you think of them in a notebook you carry in your pocket or on scraps of paper. First lines are precious and often will make the rest of the poem. They come to you as you drive, as you walk, as you think of chores, or they are triggered by emotions. You can give yourself assignments, like writing about the most beautiful vision you have ever had or the saddest. Or you can write about what is happening to you that day, what you are afraid of, what you find totally beautiful. I always have my patients look for the light in their life and write about it. I have them write about visions, transcendent experiences, religious emotions, and peace. You can always write about body feelings, pain, buzzing, energy, and expansion, or about what you see in guided imagery. As the Buddhists say, literature is the way to the mind, the way to see visions of beauty on earth.

A Story of a Man with Cancer Learning Guided Imagery

The stories patients tell are so beautiful that they become alive. Stories like this almost eclipse novels or even myths in their power and extraordinarily unique ability to touch us and heal. Michael tells this story:

One day an oncologist whom I had worked with for years called me. He told me he had referred a patient to me and he thought we would be a good match. The man was about sixty and he was a successful physician in the community. He had a good marriage and grown children and a beautiful home. He had had cancer of the colon several years before, had undergone surgery, and in the past week had had liver metastasis diagnosed. When I visited him at home, he and his wife were both there. He was recovering from a biopsy and was beginning to get his energy back. He wanted me to teach him how to use guided imagery. He had heard of it, but he had never done any inner work.

I asked him to tell me his story, and when he was telling me about finding out that the cancer had returned, his wife turned toward me and told me this story. She said that when he told her he was sick again, she had a vision. She saw herself in heaven or in a place that was not here. It was gray and had its own light coming from everywhere. She was there with her husband. She knew then that they would be together forever, that they would not be apart no matter what happened. As she told me this, she started to cry and his eyes became wet. I asked him if he felt some of this feeling, too. He told me that he saw himself with her forever, that they were like stars that were next to each other or like stars merging into one light. I asked him if he had had any other images like this, and he told me that at the beach that weekend he had seen his wife as a dolphin shining at him from the ocean. I told them that the experiences each of them had had were imagery and that all they had to do was explore the places from which these thoughts came and to look at them afterward.

The next week he told me a wonderful story. He was at the beach again, and he gave himself permission to daydream since I had told him that this was imagery. He saw his wife again as a dolphin above the ocean, and this time he called to her. She turned from a dolphin spirit into a spinning disc of many colors and spun to him. As this happened, he felt himself kissing her and merging and then the disc came into his liver and spun around and cleaned him out. I was amazed. They were sixty years old and were such beautiful lovers. Their imagery and story were of themselves as lovers together forever, and being able to merge into each other and heal each other. It was so magnificent a vision that I felt privileged to be allowed to share it with them. In his imagery he called her to him, she came as a spirit, and they merged and became one, and then she became his healing force. Seeing this vision made them both feel so much better. It gave them something to do that was deeply creative and stimulating. It took their minds off their problems and focused them on their deep love and on healing. He asked me why people had me teach them imagery when it was this easy. I told him that he was really good at it, but that some people needed help. I told him he was my teacher, that every time he told me his imagery I learned from him.

Do you daydream, do you have images of yourself that are peaceful or radiant? If you do, we invite you to have more of them as a way to get in touch with the part of you that gets ideas to write. Go to the places where this kind of imagery comes from. This is where your writing comes from, this is where your healing comes from. Remember that art, prayer, and healing all come from the same source. The imagery comes from where you make art. When you write or tell a story about light, animals, and healing, you become the story and it heals you like guided imagery. It changes your physiology to help white blood cells eat cancer cells by stimulating your brain to release neurotransmitters that activate the immune system.

Michael's Story of a Healing Journal
When Michael's wife, Nancy, was in the hospital having a bone marrow transplant for breast cancer, Michael wrote a journal. This is his story of healing himself by writing with the journal.

When Nancy was having her bone marrow transplant, I lived in her room for five weeks. She did not want me to leave her. Just the thought of me leaving triggered deep fears of being abandoned that came from her childhood when she had broken her arm and had been left in the hospital by her parents for days. I slept on a cot at her side. I called it a doggy bed, and I saw myself as a watchdog, a fierce protector and loyal constant companion. Without knowing why, I brought a borrowed laptop into the room and set up a writing studio. I knew I was going to be there for over a month, and I did this as something to keep me occupied. I had no healing intent—after all, she was the patient—and it did not occur to me that I was writing to heal myself. But I knew somehow that I had to bring in the laptop, and I did it.

After we moved into the room—which was unbelievably surreal in itself because they had told us she had a real chance of not living through the procedure—I took a table and moved it to the window and made it a desk. I put things on it that were special to me and arranged it so it felt just right. At first I could only borrow a huge portable computer (this was before the new small laptops), so I was confined to this desk studio. Each time I would sit there it was like a sacred space. It was mine; it was where I could go by myself and be inside my work. I could look out of the window and see the eucalyptus forest and the sky and the blowing San Francisco fog. I was an author, I had written fourteen books, so I was used to writing. But this was completely different. In all my previous books, I "talked" the material to Nancy and did the research, but Nancy did the writing, on the computer. Now I would be the one who wrote. Also, the books we had written were about imagery, babies, pregnancy, or disease and were always sold to a publisher in advance and written to be published. Now I was going to write only for myself. I had no goals of publishing whatever I wrote and did not censor it or criticize it at all. It was for my eyes only, and I did not care about perfection or appearing silly or happy or sad to another person.

The first day I woke up before dawn and looked around me and at first did not know where I was. I saw the room and Nancy sleeping there and I remembered what was happening and that she could die any day, and the first thing I did was start to write. What came out completely surprised me. I described the wild strangeness of coming into a hospital room with my wife of twenty-five years, and the happenings of the day in the strange world of medicine, but then I started to dream. I saw the fog comforting me, the morning light as beautiful, the sunrise as astonishing. And I saw her in bed as a woman deep in a rebirth ritual.

That shocked me, but it continued each day. I would see the room and the IV pumps, but I would also see Nancy as a spirit. I would see the nurses coming in the night as spirits. I would see the ritual-like way the procedure was moving on, and the most surprising thing is that I would pray and give thanks. For me, this was something new. I had done guided imagery with patients for years, but I had never prayed intentionally every day for healing. And in the journal on the first day, after I described what was happening, I gave thanks. I gave thanks for the beauty of the day, for the beauty of my wife, lying asleep next to me. I gave thanks for the care she was getting, and later for the journal itself, which would become my lifeline. And I prayed for my new way of seeing into sacred space.

Each time I would start to describe what was going on, it would take on the form of a shamanic story by itself. For example, the man who came to clean her room at first did not want to clean each of her frog sculptures on her altar. One day she played reggae tapes for him and he stopped. He looked around and saw the twenty feet of art on the wall, and the altar, and he looked at her. He picked up each froggy and cleaned it so softly, like a prayer. Each day from then on his cleaning of her altar became a crucial part of her health care to me. And as I wrote about it, I saw him as a protector, a cleansing force, a gentle spirit from a foreign land. In my writing, he seemed to drift in, almost not touching the earth. And Nancy would play Bob Marley's "Three Little Birds," and the refrain of "Every little ting, is gonna be all right" would roll over all of us like the early morning fog, and the room would fill with light and we would all just be in it, moving in slow motion as if in a dream. And he would look directly into her eyes and time would stop and it would be so peaceful and we were gone.

And it was the writing that let me see this illuminated reality rather than just focusing on the incredible difficulty of what was happening and its immediate real danger and darkness. That came out, too, in the journal, but it was always the brightness and the prayers of thanks that came out and transported me out of the room into a place of brilliance and vision that still amaze me even thinking about them now. I think if I had not written, I would only have seen the darkness. With the writing, I was able to cross a bridge into the light.

From Only Things of Beauty Persist, *Michael's Bone Marrow Journal*

April 1992. The human spirit is like the dawn. It comes up from the darkness, from nothingness, and floods the world with hope and joy. It dazzles us and blinds us with its first rays and reminds us that it is a new day. At dawn I opened the drapes and let in the joyful morning sun. The sky was light blue and the eucalyptus trees shimmered in the breeze. They shone with light and flashed their light green of new life back at the sun as a greeting. I put a Taize chant [sacred music sung] on the tape deck and read Julian of Norwich to Nancy. "I may make all things well, and I can make all things well, and I shall make all things well, and I will make all things well, and you will see yourself that every kind of thing will be well. You have restored my life, O God, and I wish to be in your presence." We lay together like two children waiting for their parents on Christmas morning, excited and expectant, nervous and afraid. Our love tied us together, we were as one in God awaiting the coming.

At eight in the morning a woman pushed a cart into the room and happily greeted Nancy. She said she was Joy and was "here to give you back your bone marrow." She pushed the cart across the room and started to arrange the trays and water and syringes. She poured water into the bath on top of which would defrost the marrow. I plugged the heater and motor in to warm and gently shake the water. She called a nurse and took Nancy's marrow from a small ice chest and checked each of the five small flat bags to make sure that the name and number matched Nancy's wristband. She smiled and told Nancy not to worry. She said that although it was a day filled with significance, the procedure did not hurt. She said that some people videotaped it or had family there. I had showered and combed my newly cut hair and put on a dress shirt for the occasion. The sun rose and shined into the family room where I got ready. It was like suiting up for an event, preparing for a wedding or bar mitzvah. The excitement filled the air like energy or electrons and made us both nervous. My body was shaking inside with tiny vibrations, like a taut rubber band. Joy said that this was the long-awaited day, but the procedure was not much, it was just sucking the defrosted marrow into large syringes and pushing it into Nancy's central line. . . . Thank you, Great Spirit, for your world. Thank you for this dawn and this new day. Thank you for Nancy and her life. Thank you for the doctors and nurses who care for her and their love. Help this woman, Nancy, Great Spirit, help her to live and get rid of her cancer. Give her a good life, let her be born again and be your child and be one with your world.

In this story you can see how writing heals and see the way you can easily do it yourself. All it takes is writing daily and a routine. You need a place and a habit. You need the determination and decision to write. You need to let go of judgment and self-criticism. And you just need to clear time for it and do it. The process of writing lets you see who you really are and what is important to you. All you need to do is write, and the healing happens. And it grabs you and it becomes so interesting and important that you do not have to do it with effort after a while. You do it as the first choice. It does not take much time, just a half hour or so, and you do not need much equipment or space. You just need to make the decision to go into your writing place and write for a time and then live.

For the past several years, Michael has been writing poetry each day. These poems started from the kinds of prayers and visions he first saw in his bone marrow journal. The poems bring him into a space of transcendence, which helps him deal with patients who are very ill and lets him share luminosity with them. He describes how it feels for him to write poetry now:

First I say a blessing or prayer to "Her." I close my eyes and I try to see Her in Her most magnificent aspect, as She is in this moment. Then I write down whatever comes to me without censorship. It does not have to be pretty or even poetic. It just is what comes to me clearest and is totally true. I am always surprised by what comes. It can be funny, sad, wild, astonishing. And then I start to tell the story of what is happening in the outer world to ground me, to take me from where I am now, from my lived experience. And as I write, She talks to me, and then She sings to me. She tells me who I am and She tells me how much She loves me. And as She sends me Her visions, I go deeper into the ordinary moment, the event, the actual experience that started the poem, and it turns into wonder. I fall into the moment between time and space. I can see Her dancing, I can see Her life force, I can see myself loving Her. If the poem is about shamanism, I can hear the stories of the ancient ones and the voices of the spirit animals. I can see through the eyes of the ancient ones and out of the eyes of the spirit animals. And the poem circles, spirals, whirls me deeper into Her heart, into my heart. And I see even deeper and She sings to me louder. So for me, writing is a falling, a falling into. And before I write, I quiet myself and say a prayer and ask for the truth to be told, and for my love to live forever. I do.

A STUDIO FOR WRITING

Writing requires a studio that is more in your heart than in the outer world. You can write on a pad with a pen in a break from work in one minute. The first line of a poem can come to you anywhere, and you can jot it down in a notebook wherever you are. Your studio becomes that notebook. Or you can make a whole room or even a rented space that is just yours to write healing stories in. Many writers talk about cues or habits that help them write. Writing at the same time each day, writing after a walk, in the same notebook, with the same pen, are all techniques writers use to help the words flow. Michael writes on a laptop with a painting on its case. Some writers like desks with animal fetishes, art, or music around them.

Most writers agree that it is useful to write each day for a certain period of time. This is necessary if you are trying to finish a piece, but less necessary if you are writing to heal. In writing to heal, all you need to do is let the words flow onto the paper and not censor or stop them. Let the subject be your own life as you are living it now and move from there. Don't worry about making sense or the rules of grammar or spelling, or how someone else will react to it. Write like you're making entries in a journal or composing a personal letter and let it go from there. If it turns into something you want to share or publish, great, but writing for healing is about letting your inner images be seen by you more than it is about writing a literary masterpiece.

The most basic studio is a notebook or a computer. For notebooks, you can choose one that is elaborate, with a beautiful cover, or the simplest pocket pad. You can put pictures on the cover and create collages inside with colored pens. On a computer, you can put graphics on the wallpaper backgrounds from the Internet or from purchased software that make the computer personal. Some writers make the journal or computer deeply personal, even sacred. They have a place for it in their home, they put altar figures around it, they care for it like a living thing. Whatever you do with your writing studio is fine. As you use it, you will develop a relationship to it so that it becomes like a friend or a safe place. It is the place you seek to write letters and pour out your heart. It becomes your refuge, your therapist, your lifeline.

ONCE UPON A TIME

Story time has always been outside of ordinary time and space. In fact, as any child will tell you, listening to stories takes them to a place where they lose track of time and where they seem to be somewhere else. Healing artists often say that writing takes them and their patients "elsewhere." *Else-where* means that the person's mind is off the illness, their pain decreases, their symptoms decrease, their attitude changes from fear to concentration. Stories occur in the break between moments of time and in the break between points of space. They occur in the opening into nonordinary reality. Stories often start with "once upon a time," which of course is not in ordinary time at all, and "in a far-off land," which of course is not in any place we have ever been to in the outer world.

When a story gets ancient enough it turns into a myth or legend, which means it has no known author whom anyone remembers. It has been around forever; it almost seems as if it comes from the earth. So one of the main advantages of story time is that it takes us out of ordinary time and space and into the space of myth and legend, which is precisely where we need to go to heal. Stories actually slip in between moments of time, and are in no time, and there they can live forever. And they slip in between places of space, and are in no space, and there they can move things like cancer cells away from the rules that exist in ordinary space.

Guided imagery, like story time, takes place in your imagination. Clock time does not apply in guided imagery. In fact, one hypnotic technique involves saying that "one minute of imagery time will be an hour of clock time." This would make a person feel deeply rested after only a few moments. That is how time feels to the person who is living in his or her imagination. But in story time, two more things happen that are crucial to healing. First, a person can be loved from before the beginning of time to after the end of time, for time disappears in the story. Second, people who have a life-threatening illness are not subject in their imagination to the clinical statistics that may relate to their illness.

Children live in a world that is experienced in a much different time and space, and tribal peoples live in a world where time and space are measured much differently than we measure them. The story takes us to that world, and as long as we are within its boundless realms we can create a place that is safe, where we are free. The healing artist as a storyteller takes us "elsewhere" to the nonordinary world and puts us in the realm of the miracle. Healing stories take ancient myths and make them yours. They take heroes and animal spirits and make them real to you in your life now.

Jan's Advice and Experiences

As Jan explains, a crowd of people in a hospital waiting room is a difficult audience. She comes up to them and says, "Let's tell stories, let's make art." What she invented as a storyteller was squish art. Anyone could do it. She took a little tube of paint and handed it to someone to make a painting. She would tell them to make a dot, a squirt, anything. Everyone would do it. She passed the tube of paint around. Then she would fold the paper and squish the color and she would ask, "What is it?" And then each person would answer with a story. They would see trees, landscapes, animals. There would be sudden emotion in the waiting room. Each person would tell a story about his or her own life. Suddenly the TV was background noise. Jan was so brave; she was fearless.

That is how Jan began as a storyteller. It was her entrance. She would get people to tell stories right in the waiting room. Then she would pick up her journal and sit with them in their rooms. She would transcribe their stories. As they were dying, she let them tell oral stories when they were too ill to write. They would talk, and she would transcribe for them and their families. They could call her at home. She would get involved with their lives, try to resolve their conflicts. She would be a silent witness to the stories in whatever form they would take. She followed them all the time in the hospital, from their room to their home, from admissions to discharge. For three years, she actively put this healing art into practice. She would transcribe the stories of children in the hospital. The children would write, "They said it wouldn't hurt, and it did." She got them to tell their stories and she would publish them in *Zine,* an underground hospital newspaper. She would bring stories of other children back to them, even though they did not meet each other. It was as if they wrote to each other. *Zine* came out every six weeks, networking children with their own voices.

Jan formed the Accidental Poets Society. Everyone sat and told poems on the hospital lawn. They would read their own poems, often for the first time. Many different types of artists would come and practice using poetry.

Jan advocated journal writing for all artists as healing. She saw art as "a way of living, a way of healing." This writing to heal was her life. As an artist, she got all the artists to write poetry and tell stories. She created community symposiums; she invited everyone to read the poetry, to dance and play music. She created audiences for people to read to. There was always poetry in a performance or concert. The poetry was never judged; it was just what people needed to say. She made poetry flow into the hospital like it was natural.

The most beautiful thing Jan created was herself. She created herself as a character in a novel. When she was diagnosed with pancreatic cancer, she would do visualizations, bringing her friends and artists she worked with together to ride a wave in their imagination. She would tell them, "You are on the beach with the raisin guys, with lemon slices in the surf." She had all her friends singing Beach Boy songs and doing visualizations for her. It was imagery medicine with humor, with a twist.

She always said, "Listen to what they say, let them direct you, honor the writer in everyone." Her bag was filled with notebook paper and colors to make visual journals and books for the kids she took care of. Jan said, "You know, Mary, I went to the doctor the other day. He shuffled in, he sat there and put his hands together, he said, 'The situation is very grave.' Can you believe it, he chose the word *grave*." She laughs as if it's the funniest thing she ever heard. She made her life into a story; it was hard to tell what was true and what was not true. She was persnickety, she was posed, she was dramatic. After she was diagnosed with pancreatic cancer, she eventually stopped writing in her journal. She surrounded herself with artists who would read to her, with dancers who would dance for her, with a painter who would paint for her. All the while, she was in bed at home. She created a group of people who became characters in her life. She was the author of her life. It was rich and full with music, dance, visual imagery, and, most of all, her own emerging story.

She constructed this alternative reality herself, as she would construct a story. Her husband wrote a book of poetry about it after she died. She was a living being who was the personification of a writer using writing to intentionally heal. Yet she was who she was always. She was down-to-earth, funny, spontaneous, wild. Her journal was full of her drawings, her work, her playful songs, her sensuality. The ways she used words for their sounds, their flip meanings, were never ending. She would take the truth and embellish it with imaginative details. Her descriptions made it come alive.

She had people write in a journal, in a regular notebook. In hers, she made three columns because she said it was easier to write small narrow paragraphs than larger ones. "You need only two sentences for a paragraph," she said. She wrote little pieces, she drew pictures all around the poems, she wrote in the journal every day. Sometimes she wrote paragraphs, sometimes pages. She wrote all the time. Her focus in life was to get people to write to heal.

When she became quite ill and was fighting her disease, she wrote a story of a princess who lived in a castle. She had an artist illustrate the story. She told the story as a fairy tale. She would tell the story over and over again: There was a princess who lived in a castle and was sick. (It seemed Jan was the princess.) The castle gardener was ordered to pick the flowers that were growing everywhere. The flowers were purple, and wild. The castle's gardeners picked them, and picked them, and brought them to the princess—they never could pick them all.

The story became elaborate, with many characters, which she would add to daily. She never ended it. The flowers kept growing until they took over the entire kingdom.

The story was bittersweet. Jan never said the flowers were her cancer, and she did not interpret the story at all.

Ellie's Advice on Storytelling

Ellie Sommer is the storyteller-in-residence at the University of Florida, Gainesville. She followed in the steps of Jan Swanson and has continued her programs, including the Accidental Poets and *Zine* magazine. She now has interns from the college English programs and other artists who go around with her and tell stories, draw, play music, and dance.

Ellie says:

Being a storyteller-in-residence is about getting people to tell stories. When I work with them, they can do any type of art, but storytelling is our focus. First you create a structure, then you throw away your structure. Stories are tied to all the other art forms. The visual arts or music leads to stories, dance leads to stories. Sometimes I start out with a good cliché and keep going. You try to get on a roll, have the story come out so it tumbles out. An exercise I use is to make a story from a simile, for example, "a mountain is like a _____."

I find it useful to remove myself from belief. You need to stop worrying about what makes sense. Sounding silly is all right. Let yourself sound silly, sad, whatever. When you go into a room, the parents are there and are often worried or depressed; the child is scared, sick, and away from home. I make contact with the staff; they point out the patients who need us. The staff is over-worked; they appreciate your coming. They are glad when you can make a patient feel more at ease.

Much of this work is about developing relationships with patients and staff, but sometimes it takes a while. When I enter a kid's room I often use a doll or a puppet. Kids have the imagination we have lost. We make fools of ourselves to get it back. Props, dolls, and puppets all help break the ice and are subjects for stories. Some patients will do anything; some are so ill you do everything.

You tell the story based on cues from them. Sometimes you do it all, sometimes nothing. For most of us who use verbal tools for our art, it is hard. There is a lot of censorship from your child-hood; the lessons you have had about writing papers and grades make you shy. Stories for healing do not need to make sense. Go into the world of the child, go away in four words. Make the story fun. Let the healing power of the story come from its laughter, too. The interactive story is fun. You start or they start and then the other person continues. You tell, they tell, you weave the story together or in a group. Make a story in rounds, go in a circle. Each person can make up parts of it quickly. The story takes spirals, it circles, you can see it. You can make an animal out of clay. You can then tell the story of that animal. Try to remember there are no grades in healing stories. They are healing because we allow them to be free.

HOW TO HEAL YOURSELF WITH WRITING

STEP ONE: STARTING ON THE PATH
- Take time to be with yourself to daydream.
- Create a space and a time to write.
- Value your writing time as if it were gold.
- Use a laptop computer, desktop computer, spiral notebook, or journal.
- Make a notebook your portable studio and take it everywhere.
- Write every day, a set amount of time or a set number of pages.
- Invite your muse to sing to you every day.

STEP TWO: THE JOURNEY
- Make an intention to heal yourself with writing.
- If the whole page intimidates you, write in columns.
- It might be easier to write small paragraphs or separate lines.
- Find colorful pens that delight you.
- Draw pictures along with the words.
- Decorate your computer case or journal with beautiful pictures.
- When you write, let your words flow out.
- Don't edit or censor; let go of judgment.
- Write down what you would say to someone in words.
- Don't worry about making any sense at all (think of *Finnigan's Wake* by James Joyce).
- Feel Her love surrounding you.

STEP THREE: DEEPENING
- Write every day.
- Jot down notes immediately when things come to mind.
- Bring symbols into your writing.
- Tell stories to other people out loud.
- Get into your stories; they will take you "elsewhere."
- Have conversations with your characters; invite them to appear.
- Allow yourself to flow on Her river of words.

STEP FOUR: TRANSCENDENCE

+ Tap into your soul's most powerful imagery: put it to words.
+ Find words in your writing that come up again and again: they are your themes.
+ Love your words and yourself as you read them.
+ Don't be afraid of poetry; you don't have to make it rhyme or have form.
+ Create a support group to read to one another.
+ Bring out deep memories.
+ Write a letter to yourself from your heart.
+ Let your words take you deep.
+ Make your own life Her living myth.
+ Look for images of light and joy.

THE MYSTICAL PATH: HEALING STORIES ABOUT SPRINGS AND ANIMALS

For each of us, the healing journey starts in our realization of the mystical path. There is an Indian legend that as we go through life there are always two paths that run alongside each other, like two paths running parallel across a meadow. One is the smooth or rocky path of our outer lives, and the other is the mystical inner path of the artist or healer. Before our creativity, before our healing, the mystical path emerges from the darkness across the blowing grasses and calls to us. Even before the lived experience of an illness, there is the lived experience of the glimpse of the mystical path. It is the path where we glimpse the images that will become our art, and where we will find our way to our inner artist, which in turn will lead us to our inner healer. For some of us this mystical path may have been an interest in religion, meditation, or travel. It may have been a retreat, a journey, or even a love. It often was deep in our past, and it made us who we are.

As you start to write to heal, the first thing you realize is that an ancient song is being told. This is the realization of your mystical path, your remembering. Your story will come as the story of your muse, of your inspiration, of your ancestors. The sacred spring itself, from the heart of the earth, is singing to you in the language of the healer within, in the language of the earth. In the ancient stories of artists and healers, there is the basic story of an ancient mother who has never forgotten us. This is the story that we have given you as guided imagery throughout this book. Although we have forgotten her, all she wants is to be loved, to be heard. She is the mother of us all. She whispers back to us, "It's only about loving you." In the first days of the dreamtime, she wove the threads of art and healing together. At the headspring, her spirit is seen, and this is where her spirit is strongest.

In legend, all springs on earth are connected, and the waters that flow from each of them come from the source of all the waters of the earth. The ancient woman of the springs speaks to us from each spring and—more important for writing—she speaks to us from where all springs emerge in the center of our heart. The poet and the writer are aspects of our dreaming the world. She dreams the world as she weaves. She dreams the world in spirals of ethereal beauty. The spirals rise out of her forehead as her creation. As we heal ourselves with writing, we recreate her path by telling stories on her sacred spiral. We go inside and go deeper and deeper within ourselves in a spiral movement. The spirals grow and take us further and we see, we change, we grow, and we heal. The spirals, her spirals of creation, become our spirals of art and healing. The sacred spiral becomes a creative spiral that is all of our energies spun together to heal the earth. Part of this work is to remember the creative ways of being, to remember our own wildness, the untamed part of ourselves that we have evolved away from, the spirit of the ancient woman in the spring. She sings. Do you hear her song?

For this chapter on writing and storytelling, we will tell a story from legends that talk about the springs in Native American terms. This story is about the old woman of the springs as a medicine woman. In this story, she was the woman who gave birth to the spirit animals. In art and healing, almost all artist healers use animals as subjects of art. The dancer Anna Halprin has all of the people she dances with dance as an animal because she believes it brings out memories of power and strength that cancer patients need in order to heal. Patients have animals at their bedside—stuffed animals, sculptures, Zuni fetishes. Animals have a primal energy that empowers us in our healing. Here is an old story of the ancient woman of the springs creating the spirit animals.

I will tell you a story, the story of the old woman of the springs and the creation of the medicine wheel. One day she was deep in her dream; she was painting the earth into being, she was dreaming your joy into your soul. And she sings to you, she sings of the creation, she does. Now we are listening for the voices to be heard in the beauty of the day, in the dark of the night, in the crystal of the dawn. The oldest story of creation, of the medicine wheel itself, comes from her. It comes from the ancient culture that rests as a dream outside of us and inside of us at once. It comes out of who we are as the people of this land. It comes from the springs itself; it comes from the voices of the animal spirits. They all tell us of an ancient woman who is dreaming us all, who sits on the side of a spring. She still in this very moment of this very breath weaves the threads of art and healing, and they are connected to us. The silver and golden threads go right to our hearts. They are our remembrance, our dreams, our heritage.

They say that in the beginning, in the void of silence where everything is about to be born, is the place in all of us that is eternal spaciousness, the place where the ancient ones recede to. In our inner world, it is empty, it lies in nothingness. It is the home of the lost stories, of the intangible. It is there that she is dreaming. She sits on the edge of the river, right within the very source of things, before the beginning of the cycles, with the ancient turtle, the snake, the water animals, with water itself. She is a mystery; she is unending; she is connected to all things. She is the place from which we all were born, from which we were dreamed, even before the one became two. The place where they were one, where they were everything and nothing, before they were separated.

She is an eternal guardian of our dreams, our creativity, and our lives. She had been weaving the dream of art and healing as one from before eternity. She is the mother of all mothers, born from

that place coming to us as a silver thread in a spiral spinning forever. Somewhere along the spiral there is matter. Somehow
along the spiral there is you. We are born into collective community; the medicine wheel of the four directions and their animals is the earth's voice, the voice of the earth from ancient
tradition, where there was no separation of humans from animals. It was before separateness. It was within oneness, before
you could look at another and know you are not her. We forget
this separate place when illness occurs. We fall back into place,
into oneness, to heal. On the side of the sacred river she dreams
us and connects us back to the other vision.

She weaves the two energies of art and healing, of man and
woman, of light and darkness, of thinking and feeling. And the
ancient woman of the medicine wheel dreams the spirit animals
into being. She has woven the opposites together forever. She
tells us the story of the medicine wheel. She tells us the story
through the animals. The animals tell it, the art tells it, the visions
tell it. The spirit animals are the story. The owl of the east tells
you of the dawn. The owl tells you about the air and about
change. The lion of the south sings of the fire and about the passion. The bear of the west tells of healing, about water, about
where images come from. The turtle of the north tells us about
grounding, about your family, job, about the earth.

The ancient woman weaves the sacred medicine wheel in silence.
We are being dreamed by her as a dreamer. We bring art and
healing together as one. We go toward this dream in our love spiral.
Together we weave it, and spiral it out. We go into the meadow
and fall into the vortex for a hundred years. The owl calls, the lion
roars, the bear growls, the turtle swims; we hear it and tell its story.
In her world of the deep dream, she created the spirit animals first.
She gave them voices and she let them sing. They created the
directions and time and space and then, finally, the earth.

HOW ART AND HEALING CAME APART

The oldest stories and songs of the ancient healers tell us that in the beginning of time, art and healing were one. They were one being, one energy, one ancient living creature. They were one way before space and time, long before matter. And then they came apart four times. Each time they came apart, they were more and more separate. First they were just not one, later they were two, later they didn't even touch, and even later they couldn't see each other. But that is our story, that is what we will tell you. It comes from an ancient tribal song, whose author is long forgotten. It has been told and retold in many traditions. It appears in folktales, Judaism, Sufi tales, and songs.

> Once, deep in the before, art and healing were one. They were one like the sea of milk, they were one like God, they were one like Her breath. When art and healing were one, there was nothing else; there was no time and space, no directions, no past, present, or future, no large or small, no creator or created, no nothing. There was only the one, the everything, the incomparable, the always, the rest. Some say that the one never sleeps but was meditating forever on pure love, and some say that the one has no characteristics at all and cannot even be seen, felt, or spoken about. In any case, the one was also art and healing as one, for it was everything as one. And when the one became two, art and healing also became two, for everything was the same in the first breath. And when one became two, everything became two. So the first time art and healing came apart, they separated only to see each other and make the four directions. Then time and space were born and matter was formed and the stars themselves were born. At that moment, art and healing came apart again, too.
>
> Then, many years went by, and the animals were born and then the people were born. And the people saw art and healing as one; they saw spirits all around them, and they were at one with their world. When people started to work and grow crops, many of them stopped seeing the spirits and stopped making art, and

art and healing separated for the third time. Then, thousands of years went by, and time was moving fast and space was larger and science was born and modern medicine was born and hospitals were born and we are in the present time. Now the body is seen as only molecules and art is for sale and collected and hung on walls and in museums. Art and healing separated for the fourth time when medicine stopped believing in the mind or spirit and in meditation or prayer as healing. Now art and healing could not even see each other across the room.

But many people knew that a prophecy foretold that now is the time on earth for art and healing to come together again. It had long been told that now is the time this conjunction needs to be made for each of us. People knew that they needed to do creative healing now. They knew that it was imperative to do this now for the healing of the health-care system and their own personal lives. Now is the time for the artist and healer to rejoin as one. Now is the time for the rejoining of the two energies. And art and healing saw each other across the room. They came together as if they had been apart for a million years. They merged and vibrated as one. The one that separated into two had come back together as one. Time and space were here and not here at once, and the earth was healed.

In this story, art and healing are like incarnations of two energies—male and female energy, light and dark, positive and negative, yin and yang, active and passive, penetrating and receiving, wisdom and compassion, the creative and the receptive—that balance each other, that by their very existence hold the universe together and keep it alive. Whenever we talk about art and healing becoming one, we also talk about the male and the female energies and all the other energies joining and coming together to be one. So in this story, art and healing find each other and live happily forever. It has a happy ending. As you use art to heal yourself, you bring the two sides together inside you and you are one. That is how you change, that is how we heal, that is how the earth is healing herself.

John Graham-Pole, M.D., Talks about Poetry, Laughter, and Healing
John Graham-Pole is a pediatric oncologist, a poet, and a clown. He cofounded the Arts In Medicine program at the University of Florida, Gainesville, with Mary Rockwood Lane. Poetry helps him be himself and helps him deal with the serious illnesses of the children he takes care of. It calms him, helps him see the children as beautiful, and helps him continue his work without burning out. Being a clown helps him bring laughter to the kids and staff. He teaches "laughter and play" workshops to show nurses and physicians how to make patients laugh and how to bring laughter into their own lives. Here is a poem he wrote about a patient he was taking care of.

Cell Shed
Our cells
mingle, shed in
spindrift of water—
air between our
mouths. Each with
each other's tissue. You
dying, take my
part to rest.
I, living,
imbibe,
scatter your
seed.

This is a way of looking at a patient that is profoundly different. It brings the physician into a way of seeing and relating that is the way of the artist. The physician poet sees beauty and merges with the patient. His care and his way of being as a healer are changed forever. John write poems anywhere. He pauses in the hospital to write after he sees a patient. He writes in a small notebook, jotting down first lines of poems in the hall. John says that the poems help him see differently and take care of patients in a more intimate way, perceiving each person as uniquely human and not just as a case. He sees beauty in very dark situations and can handle it much better because of his poetry.

EIGHT

Healing Yourself with Movement: Dance as Healing

This chapter brings movement and beauty into your life. The dancer-in-residence will invite you to dance. As you read this chapter take the opportunities that occur in your everyday life and feel the grace and beauty as your body moves through space and time. You will become the dancer and your life will become a dance. In the sharing of the following stories, the dancers-in-residence give you voices of encouragement to use movement in your creative healing journey.

INTRODUCING YOUR DANCER-IN-RESIDENCE

The dancer walks gracefully into the patient's room. She is how you imagined a dancer would be: ethereal. She enters the cool, sterile, mechanical world of an intensive-care unit. On the white-sheeted bed, the child stirs. He is isolated, weak, and sick. She glides over to him, asks him if he would like to choose a favorite music; she'll dance with him. He pauses, hesitant about this unusual request, but he is curious, yearns for life, for lightness, for healing. He looks up at her; maybe she will dance. And she does, amidst the IV poles and monitors and multiple vials and tubes filled with his many medications.

Within this tiny sterile hospital room, cluttered with the hospital machinery of our times, she dances. And gradually she brings the child into the movement; at first he follows her just with his eyes. Then he reaches up, his outstretched arms grasp her hands, responding to her invitation. They hold each other, begin to sway . . . begin to dance together. "Welcome," she says, as she moves softly, like the mists. "I am Jill. I am a dancer. I will dance for you."

Jill Sonke Henderson is the dancer-in-residence at Shands Hospital at the University of Florida's Arts In Medicine program and the founder and director of the Dance for Life program at the University of Florida. She is one of the premier dance healers, and just watching her work is a great gift.

HOW DANCE HEALS

Dance for healing is about moving. With every movement, you embody the creative fire. There, within the dance, your body has a life of its own. Within every one of us is a dancer. The dancer within us is the seducer, the seductress, the one who creates a healing spiral around us. If we are seduced enough, we move into the dance and become part of the movement of healing. If you are a nurse, a mother, a person who is ill, you start to dance from room to room. You are in the midst of tasks, and if, within all of this, you close your eyes and see yourself as a dancer, you see that you live in the dance of your own life. Instead of rushing from place to place, you shift your body's perspective. All of a sudden, you see yourself dancing through your own life. You become graceful and beautiful by a deliberate, conscious act, an intention.

Through this possibility of dancing at any moment in our lives, dancing *in* any moment, we can see ourselves in total grace and beauty. In the dancing moment there is a level of spontaneity and fun. You can move in any way you want to. You dance and twirl, allow yourself to stretch, to open. Embody movement that is natural and flowing, like a river. Your movements become art; they become a dance.

Dance heals by spiraling us down inside ourselves to a center where tensions are released and there is freedom and spaciousness. To dance is to harness the fire inside your belly that moves you. You are always in movement; you go inside where you are held in place and then move outward. You thrill to the momentum and the movement that frees you. You feel the wind as you move; it enlivens your senses. You twirl, you move, you feel your spirit's rhythm.

Dance is a vehicle for emotional expression, an opportunity to embody emotion. When she teaches, Jill has people dance an image of a scene, become a forest, an animal. Each person chooses an image and dances it to another person. Then they dance together. Then Jill has people dance a moment of pain or illness. She uses the dance as a way to connect to someone. You can become sensitive to how you move and how another person moves. You move with them and let them push on your hand. You connect with the essential energy all people have inside themselves. Each person has a specific energy, a way of moving. You connect with it and harness it for healing. You start to move, you get into your energy, you get tingly, alive. Your cells vibrate; you tap into your own energy source. As you move, you feel the imagery within you become real, you feel it become alive. If you imagine you are a tree, you move your arms as branches and you feel like a tree. When you dance with someone who is ill, your very movements flow to them—lift them or caress them and send them your healing energy.

All the imagery does is take you into the dance. What is healing is the actual dance. Your body and spirit become one and really free. The energy of the experience becomes palpable. Writing, painting, song, and dance are like a continuum that goes from thought to movement, embodying the creative process. In dance, you are truly embodied, translating thought and emotion into movement. When you get cells moving, neurotransmitters flow, endorphins flow. You express any fluidity you are capable of. Whatever is tense is let go. The body itself leads you to where it wants to be naturally.

How does it feel to experience creative healing, to be within the creative fire? This is one dancer's experience of being an artist healer working with patients.

As I go deep into the sacred spiral, as I fall deeply into the center of the spiral of art and healing, through my love and through my dreams of creation itself, I fall into the center of the spiral nebulus and this is what I see: there is a moment where the artist and healer are one. It may simply be the moment when they are one with their own inner artist or with the artist in the room with them. In that moment, magic happens. The creative process, the same process that fuels the universe, that causes stars to be born, spiral nebula to come, babies to be born, also heals cells and changes a person forever. I get a feeling of deep peace. My body is calm and electric at once. I see everywhere. I am connected to everything. The release of the inner imagery from the creative source changes the person's life and body; it heals the person.

But what actually happens in this moment of dance as magic? What is the actual process by which prayer or mind-body connections or creativity heals? We believe it is the same process in which the universe is formed from the dream, that matter is formed from thought. Just as the universe is creative by making stars, you are creative by dancing. We believe the process is the same. As you explore the artist within, you will connect to the deepest moments in your life. It is this deeper place of being where you'll find inner peace.

JILL'S ADVICE ABOUT USING DANCE TO HEAL YOURSELF: MAKING A DANCE STUDIO

You need to create an environment that is supportive of the kind of work you want to do. It is important that the world around you support you and recognize you. Making a studio creates a tangible way for you to be seen as an artist—both in your own eyes and in the eyes of others. It focuses your mind on who you are and what you are trying to become. You may be blocked now by your fear of not doing art right, but if you do it every day you will be the artist you want to be. Create the space and your form will follow you.

Jill started out not knowing what to do. She rented a place where she could dance, and she stood in the middle of the dance floor not knowing what she was going to do to start. First she danced a few steps, then a few more; then she did workshops, then she realized that she believed the process was healing. Now she dances every day in the hospital and runs the Dance for Life program in Arts In Medicine. It all started with her renting a new studio.

You can dance in any space. If you make a space your own, it becomes your sacred studio and the place that triggers your shift in consciousness. In the space, put materials that are useful for dancing. I use silk scarves, which can be bought from suppliers, secondhand shops, and discount stores or found in your own attic or closet. I also use fabric of all colors and shapes. The scarves and fabric are the costumes or props. They transform you into what you are dancing. For example, if you dance the waters of the spring, flowing blue scarves make you the swirling water. I also use magic feathers from crafts shops and magic wands made from dowels wrapped in ribbon. The wands can have streamers and glitter or anything you like on them. Like the scarves, they add to the costume and make you embody what you are dancing.

I carry a selection of tapes of classical, piano, new-age instrumental, and children's instrumental music. I also have tapes of the environment—ocean, rain forest, etc. I also have musical instruments such as drums, shakers, a lap harp, sticks, and bells. In addition, I carry art supplies such as crayons, paper, paints, markers, glue, scissors, ribbon, glitter, and materials for making jewelry. These are the same types of supplies used for visual arts. In dance, I use them to enhance the costume and the setting. You can make sets that become the dancer's world. Socks can be used for making puppets; face paint and jewels can also help people be what they are dancing.

To begin to dance we first must find a starting place. I ask the patients about what activities they enjoy. What is their favorite thing to do? What are they experts in? What is important in their lives? What are they proud of? For patients who are ill, it is very useful to ask what they would like to be doing instead of being in the hospital. What are their fondest dreams? Or what images keep coming up in dreams that they remember? What do they love or miss about home or some place special? What do they want to do when they are well?

If people have already been involved in art, I ask them about the process in detail. If they are not forthcoming, I try to get them to talk while we paint. I can often tell where to start by just looking around their room and seeing what is hung there, what they have been sent. Sometimes just moving or doing imagery helps us find significant images to dance to.

You also can start to dance with pure movement explorations. Move as if you are in an environment, as if you are something—an animal, flower, water. Move as if you were made of clay or wax. Pretend you are doing something like catching a ball. Imagine you are in a space like a bubble. Move to define the space. Move to fill an imaginary empty vessel. Move your body to get in touch with your breath, your blood, your heartbeat.

Imagery is an important part of the healing dance process. Moving from images is an important part of dancing to heal. You can find personal images through any of the processes above or you can do guided imagery exercises to find healing images to dance to.

Jill says that for her, dancing takes her into herself. There she spirals into her spirit and can use the energy to pick up a child with cancer and lift that child upward. Jill's story illustrates many of the points of healing yourself with dance. As a dancer-in-residence for four years, she has learned much about healing dance that is useful to us, so we will tell her story in detail.

An Interview with Jill Sonke Henderson

I started dancing at seventeen. Once I discovered dancing, I danced every day. I knew I had to do it. At twenty-one, I went to Interlochen Arts Academy and Florida State University, where I majored in dance, then to New York to dance professionally. Then I got sick. I came down initially with herpes and was really sick in bed for three weeks. I was in too much pain to move. I found myself turning on the classical radio station and just letting it play all day. I would just lie on my back and visualize myself dancing to the music. I would get way inside the music and inside my body, visualize, and dance all day. I was energetically alive, even though my body just wanted to die. I was in a lot of pain. I had about fifty lesions and was throwing up. I didn't want to be in that body at all, but deeper inside it was really light and I could do anything I wanted with my body in imagery. I could feel the energy stirring inside me.

I still see energy this way. Like when you're sleeping, your cells are moving really slowly and you wake up and your cells move a little quicker and something excites you and they move faster and faster and when you get your own physical movement in it everything just swirls and swirls and swirls. I could feel that when I was just lying there. I could feel that energy swirling, and it felt really alive and wonderful. It was just a tremendous experience. It was like being out of my body, even though I was just lying there still. I was aware that the pain and the discomfort were there, but I was so far inside my body that I could feel my body in the movement and I could do anything I wanted with it. I could bend it in ways I normally couldn't bend it. I had complete freedom. It was like feeling great inside this body that felt like shit. I loved that experience, even though I didn't think much of it in terms of its value at that time. I remember how incredibly helpful it was. I think it helped the healing in that the energy was moving inside me, causing flow, instead of me just feeling that nothing was moving.

I couldn't dance for a while. It took a while for me to get my energy back—about a month and a half. That was the first experience I had of leaving dance, having an intense life experience, and then coming back to it. Every time that's happened in my life, I come back and I feel like it just enhances my dance so much. I come back and I don't feel like, "Oh, my God, I'm out of shape and it's going to take me months to get back to the level I was at." I feel like I come back a better dancer every time. My structure and my value system concerning dance might be different from a ballet dancer's. If my leg only goes up to here instead of here I don't feel like I'm a worse dancer. But if my emotional connection to my dance and my accessibility to my inner self is clearer and more available, I feel like I'm a better dancer. It might be a little different for me than for other dancers.

I have always had an attraction to being a health-care giver, and my whole process with dance was deepening. When I dance sometimes and I'm just riding on the music, the stuff that doesn't need to be there flies off, flings off, and it gets clearer and lighter and cleaner and you get inside and then whoosh! You find that place that is just free. Freedom, just space—no time—it's just space and it's just energy and then you ride it, just spiraling colors and lights. I knew that if I could facilitate a process like this for patients, it could be very helpful and healing.

It was never there until I walked from the art studio into the first patient's room, there by myself. As I walked down that hall, I had no idea what to do, and somewhere between here and there I thought, "Okay, I'm going to fly paper airplanes." So that's what we did and it worked. It bridged us beautifully into movement and of course he was wide open and he was just a perfect, perfect person to be that first patient. It was on the bone marrow transplant unit, and he was five years old. Each patient on this unit is in isolation, living in a confined space, with multiple IV medications on poles. This process takes place in an intensive-care unit, usually in a hospital bed or on a blanket spread

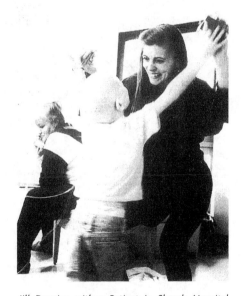

Jill Dancing with a Patient in Shands Hospital. Within this tiny sterile hospital room, cluttered with the hospital machinery of our times, she dances. And gradually she brings the child into the movement; at first he follows her just with his eyes. Then he reaches up, his outstretched arms grasp her hands, responding to her invitation. They hold each other, begin to sway, and they begin to dance together.

on the small floor space. He was there with his mom and dad, who were wonderfully supportive. They were ready to do anything he wanted to do. His room, like all the rooms there, was very small. There's the bed, the chair, the stool, and the poles, and there's just room to maneuver around those things. If you push the furniture to the sides, which we did, and tape a blanket to the floor, it gives you maybe a four- to five-by-six-foot area to move in, which for him was plenty.

So that first day we made paper airplanes and we decorated them and started flying. I had been oriented to the intensive-care unit, so I knew most of the safety things that you have to know, but I didn't know that he couldn't touch the floor; things couldn't touch the floor. His parents very kindly cued me in to that as I was guiding him to the floor at one point. We had our airplanes decorated to fly, and I just said, "Where do you want to go?" He said, "To the mountains." So we flew to the mountains in our airplane, going up and down. Knowing that he had been in his bed for quite a long time, I was trying to give him a range of physical movement. So we were flying over the mountains and spiraling down.

He had just had his transplant. He was probably half a week beyond it. So as we flew, he'd start crushing the mountains and knocking them down and then suddenly he'd go and he'd run and hide. We'd just have to hide and wait quietly for a few minutes, then he'd go crush the mountains again. Then we pretended to fly to New York and we smashed buildings and knocked them down. It was real determined, aggressive stuff, but we'd always stop and hide for a while. He'd be moving with me. We'd be going together. We'd be squatting down, walking in a squat across the room and then reaching up to the ceiling and then dropping down quickly and he'd be stomping on the mountains and smashing them with his hands and jumping and screaming and being really verbal.

He liked drumming music, so I'd bring in tapes to give us a beat. I'd just name movement elements like running, jumping, turning, shaking, stretching, reaching, whatever. There was only one rule: you couldn't do any of those like you normally do. You had to do them differently. You could be crazy, you could be silly, you could be anything, but if you were going to walk you had to walk with an elbow in the air, with your head dropped over, or some different way with everything. So it was like a stop-freeze game. I'd say "Freeze!" and make a funny shape and then we'd see how many different ways we could shake different parts of our bodies, and this was all to the music. He'd connect nicely to the music. We'd walk and run and jump and turn, and although he could only turn three-quarters at a time because of his IV lines, his parents and I would try to give him as much physical freedom as possible, grabbing the lines around so he could move.

The next day, I asked if he'd like to play a game. He could be anything he wanted to be, a creature, an alien, an animal, anything real or imagined, and right away he knew he wanted to be a dragon. So I brought in a T-shirt and a hat and we started making his dragon costume and I was amazed at how clear he was. He knew his dragon had purple paws with gold toes and it had a purple diamond on its chest. Everything was really specific—he knew exactly what he wanted. We took this hat—you know, one of those fold-up sailor hats—and dropped the front down and cut eye holes so he could make a mask, and this was like a full dragon costume. He was this dragon, again crushing mountains and fighting battles. And then his mom and I became his footmen to help him. He'd show us how to hit, how to do everything, and we started helping him. We all wore masks. He totally directed the story at this point. He was directing almost from the beginning. Starting with the battle stuff, he'd give us our instruments. Mine was like this, two fingers sticking out, my arm straight. His mom was holding a sword. We'd each have to punch a certain way and he'd say, "Okay, there are thirty-seven warriors, we have to get them." He'd be the main dude; we'd only get to kill a few. So we just fought battle after battle after battle.

For anybody interested in dance, we advise that you stretch and warm up, but then do improvisational things where you just move. If you are working with others, have a lot of contact. Use a lot of images, sacred images, starting with a simple sequence of movements. Say you're going to enter this space holding an object or holding something in your hands that's symbolic to you. It can be a golden sphere of light. It can represent something you want to give up—something you want to give to the universe. It can represent what you have to offer the world. It can be anything; just let it represent something for you. Take it into this space, offer it up, and then release it. Then come down to the earth in some way just to receive the energy of the earth.

> I think there's a space that's palpable. Being on this unit, I do my best to create sacred space and to be really intentional about walking into a room. You can walk into a room and the energy will feel different; you know, it just feels different. It's a different plane, a different level of being. The person in the room and his or her support people—they're living differently. They're not dressing, they're not doing, they're not in the world in that way at all. They're just focused on their process for the most part. Of course, sometimes you get people who don't go into a deep inner process even in this life-and-death situation. But this space changes. When a patient is embracing or engaging in a creative process, the room changes. If I had to describe in words the quality of the space, it would be almost like the air is thicker, more like fluid. There's more vibration in my body. I'm definitely more in the moment. There's not much mind chatter—I'm more in my body. And I can feel it when I leave the room and feel the space change. I can still feel my body vibrating differently.

The Story of Anna Halprin: Healing Her Own Cancer with Dance

Anna Halprin is the grandmother of healing dance and one of the most stellar pioneers in the field of art and healing. At the time of this interview she was seventy-five years old and had just won a lifetime dance career award. She is a small woman with a body that looks as if it can move in every way. Her pelvis is as flexible as a young dancer's is, and she laughs, cries, smiles, and engages you with her eyes and personality. When she talks about dance and healing, you feel as if you are hearing someone whose depth of knowledge is ancient and profound. Here she tells her story of how she healed herself of cancer with dance.

As a dancer working from a holistic approach, I have always been concerned with the relationship between the mind and the body. Understanding the connection of movements with feelings is easy enough, but understanding how the mind works in relation to the body isn't that simple. I was exploring the use of imagery as a way of making that link. I found it wasn't enough to create images in the mind's eye; I wanted people to draw their own images, reflect upon them, and learn physically the language of these images. The process of connection with our internal imagery involved "dancing" the images that welled up from this unconscious as another way of connecting the mind and the body. In learning this imagistic language, it became clear I was receiving messages from an intelligence within the body, an intelligence deeper and more unpredictable than anything I could understand through rational thought.

While I was participating in this PsychoKinetic Visualization Process, I drew an image of myself that I was unable to dance. This was a signal to me. Why couldn't I dance? What was blocking me? I had drawn a round ball in my pelvic area, and I intellectualized that it was pointing a way to new beginnings. But some part of me was sure that this approach to my drawing was nonsense, because I wouldn't be able to put the drawing into motion. That night, when my mind was quiet, I had intimations that the image I had drawn had something to tell me, and that I was not listening.

The next day I made an appointment with my doctor. I asked him to examine me precisely where I had drawn this round ball. He diagnosed cancer. I went though the traditional operation procedures—and radical ones at that—which altered my body for life, leaving me with a colostomy and feelings of real uncertainty about my future. Would I ever dance again? The doctor assured me I was just fine, which was funny because I didn't feel fine. He added that if I didn't have a recurrence within five years, I would be totally out of the woods. Three years after my operation I had a recurrence. I knew then that I was going to have to make some very drastic changes in my life.

After my recovery from the operation, I began intensive research. I wanted to understand how it was possible to receive an unconscious message about something in the body through a drawing. For a period of three years, I collected slides of drawings done by students in my classes, and I studied them, trying to find a coherent visual language I could understand. I thought perhaps certain colors or shapes meant something, or that certain symbols had a particular meaning. But if there was a system in this, I could not find it. What I did find was that none of these questions could be answered in a rational, logical, or systematic manner. It just didn't work that way. What seemed to work was the process; when people danced their images and moved back and forth between dancing and drawing, the messages would be made clear through the movements and drawings. The visual images couldn't be codified in rigid terms because each person had their own unique story, expressed in their own personal way.

At the same time, certain symbols and principles seemed to repeat themselves. For example, in a whole classroom of self-portraits, you might notice that almost everyone had a snake or a tree or a water image in their drawing. Or that the drawings indicated polarities or opposites—a dark and a light side. In conjunction with the intense individuality of the drawings, I saw certain common themes repeated over and over again. I also learned that until these images were personally experienced through dance and movement, their messages remained mysterious. I began to suspect that some of the repeating images and polarities had to do with the ways we are all connected to our common environment, the natural world, and the elements that make all our lives similar to one another's.

Let me give an example of how I was able to learn something about my own life story, the mystery of my own personal imagery, and my connection to the natural world by dancing a self-portrait I did at the time of my illness. When I first drew myself, I made myself look "perfect." I was young and brightly colored. My hair was blowing in the wind. I was the picture of health and vitality. When I looked at the picture after drawing it, I knew I couldn't even begin to dance it; it just didn't feel like me. I turned the paper over and furiously began to draw another image of myself. It was black and angular and angry and violent. I knew that this backside image of me was the dance I had to do.

I stood there, and I looked at it. To get started, I took the position I'd drawn, the position of this person with a knife in her hand and the hand up. So I stood in that position with my hand poised like this. Immediately my muscles had to tighten to hold onto the knife, and as my hand tightened to hold onto the knife it became a fist and that fist and that muscular contraction immediately set off a response of anger. I mean, if you were holding a knife in your hand and it was pointing toward your body, it would set off anger. It also set off rage and hysteria because it was aimed at me, so it was as if I was stabbing and killing myself. It was the worst kind of demon image that was coming into me, and the moment I started, it just took over.

Now, when I danced it physically, I went into a rage. I started talking in what people call "tongues." It was incoherent, but I was just screaming these words. I had no idea what they meant and I was stabbing at myself and I was so angry that I don't even know what I was doing. When I looked at the videotape, I could just feel this anger bottle up. Usually when I dance, I know what I'm doing. I can shape my movement and I know how I can develop the movement. I'm very much a skilled technician developing my material as it comes out, like a painter would see the painting in front of them and then develop it. Well, I can do that with movement, because that's what my skill is. But when I was doing this there was no such connection, there was no ability to impose an aesthetic shape. Whatever came out was just explosive—kind of out of control. This was unusual for me, so in a sense, I think of it as an exorcism rather than as any kind of aesthetic dance. The sounds, too, just came.

That was the starting point. The moment I took that first "explosion" of sound, I embodied my own demon. Once it started, it was thoughtless; it was movement, straight movement. And that's when the release happened. I was exhausted, I was just physically exhausted. I got to a point where I didn't have any more energy. I was just exhausted. And if you see the tape, it's not an aesthetic. If I were to do this as a dance, I would have developed the material very differently.

Oh yeah, that's what I felt. Well, you can see in the dance that I just fall onto my knees. I didn't just collapse. I felt the kind of tears that were connected to a very, very deep sadness. But at the same time, it was a release, and that's when I fell, and that's when I felt my diaphragm just breaking. The tears were just the inner sensation of this dam of water, and the breath was like water. It started in my diaphragm and it just burst forth, and my whole body just melted, just softened, and I just sobbed and sobbed and cried. And it was a very strong physical sensation. The demon within me certainly had a long history. I felt that it came from a very ancient place. It felt very ancient. The way I drew myself, I felt like a female warrior.

Do you know what I think happened, in retrospect? I think that when this diaphragm felt like it was a dam and it had broken and the water started rushing, I think that in retrospect that was the turning point. I think that something was released. I don't know if it was on an herb-assisted level, a chemical level, or an electrical level, but I suspect something because of the intensity of the sensation—I mean, I could not have stood up at that point. It was just flowing. I could not feel anything at that moment. It was its own movement. You couldn't see it, but if you look at the video, you could just see my back.

I felt when this thing opened up here and started flowing down that I was on earth and that it was flowing into the earth; the water that was coming through me was just flowing through me into the earth. I felt so connected to the earth. I was this demon. It was very real, but it wasn't me in this world. It may have been just this intense fantasy that came from the drawing, but when I let go I was no longer a human form. This water just took over and I was part of the earth and when I stood up and turned around, I started dancing, I was just dancing my breath because I had just let it out. I was just breathing and my breath was water. I felt like I was washing myself, just cleansing myself with this water, and the movements were water movements— very fluid water movements. That image of the breath and water is something I use to this day if something's wrong. Once I had a lecture to give and I had laryngitis, and I spent the whole day just imagining that there was this waterfall and it had mossy green stuff on it and clean water was just going through my throat, and that night I was able to give the lecture, but the next day the laryngitis came back. So in the second dance, where it turned around, I was a human form.

I had to have witnesses, because I knew unless I did, I would never be able to go though this ordeal. My witnesses were my family, colleagues, and my students, and they kept me honest, urging me to go deeper, reinforcing my sounds, calling out parts of the picture I was to dance. I danced until I was spent, and I collapsed and I began to sob with great relief. Now I was ready to turn the picture over and dance the healing image of myself.

As I danced this image, I imagined that my breath was water and that my movements flowed though my body just as water would flow. I imagined the water was cleansing me. I had an image of water cascading over the mountains near my home, and that water flowed through me and out to the endless vastness of the sea, taking with it my illness. I believe I was experiencing the forces of nature as they are imprinted into my body, which gave me a deep sense of the real connection between my body and the world around me. The movements of this dance started soft and small, and as I continued to dance, I added sound. My witnesses again reinforced these sounds, as the movements grew and grew, until my whole body was engaged in the image of cascading waters. When I finished, I invited the witnesses to join me in a circle; I felt ready to return to my friends and family.

Something happened to me in this dance that I can't explain. I felt I had been on a mysterious journey to an ancient world. Time and place were suspended and I was in a timeless blue void. The experience left me trembling and purified. Later, as I gained distance from the experience of my dance, I began to notice a pattern within it that seemed relevant to other healing processes. I have mapped out the touchstones of that journey.

The first was to simply look and identify the issue, the polarity between the dark side and the light side. The second point in my journey was the actual confrontation, which was followed by a release. After the release, the third task was finding some way to integrate the new changes in my body. That's what I did when I did the water dance. The last step in the journey was assimilation, a coming back to my community and my family and my life.

Much later, when I was developing a theory and methods to apply to my teaching, I saw how this experience was the source of a healing process I had begun to identify. This experience gave me a new way of looking at healing, which I have used ever since as a guide to working with others. I call this process the Five Stages of Healing and have adapted it to working with other people with life-threatening conditions and larger community contexts in the form of ritual and group healings. In 1981, I began to apply this process to a whole community of people. I began to create large-scale rituals that addressed the different needs of the communities with which I worked, and I always applied this process of drawing and dancing as a way to generate what I call resources.

I am so captivated by the discoveries that happen in the visualization process and in this road map for the healing journey that I often forget to tell my friends and readers that after this dance my cancer went into a spontaneous remission. It is the healing process implicit in this journey that interests me as much as the cure, because healing is a whole process available to all of us, all the time. A cure is an event, neither predictable nor always available. The process of healing rests within dance, an ancient practice with wonderful possibilities for us today.

An Interview with Anna about Healing Dance

I have people start out with something very simple and basic, and then I usually have them work with their eyes closed. I just empathize and watch and see where they take that material. I might draw out an image, or I might get an idea for an image from empathizing with somebody. I trust the process so thoroughly that I really give people whatever time they need, and I trust that if they stay with their eyes closed and with the sensation of the movement that it will take them somewhere. I just see where it's going by feeling it myself with them, and then, very often, I find that when the group can connect with other people or even one or two people that this will bring them to another level of the depth of their experience. I like to just keep making the connections broader and broader until, if possible, the whole group will come together in the connection. Every time a new connection is made, it seems like it intensifies their own experience. Sometimes they'll dance, sometimes somebody will make a sound in one corner and somebody will echo it in the other corner, and then, even though their movements are separate, they feel the voices. Sometimes someone's movement will swirl around them and that will catapult them to another level.

One woman had never danced before, and she had been telling us how she had been struggling with cervix cancer and how it had metastasized and she just felt so hopeless and so depressed. When I saw her doing her movement—she just got swept into it—I empathized with her and I said, "Oh, this is good, I want to support her." I said to myself, "I'm going to get these cancer cells together—I'm going to get them out and I'm mad and I'm angry." You can't be depressed and do a movement like that. The anger will give you some motivation—some life force. If you get into angry feelings, just think about the pure energy of your feelings. I just give them permission to do anything. Anything they do is going to be okay. If they're doing it, it's because they need to do it. So there's a lot of permission.

I am so open and accepting and I'm so totally nonjudgmental. Last night when this woman was telling us about how depressed she was, everybody was trying to fix it, you know, and I let them do that and then I just started dancing it. I said, "You really feel shitty?" "Yeah, I feel shitty." I said, "What the hell, how would you—if you couldn't say it in words—how would you say it in movement?" She went, "Yeach!" and we all did the same, and before you know it the whole class was doing that and because she was able to express it, she started laughing, she started smiling. So I think that what happens is that the group feels they can trust me, that I'm not going to take over, that I'm not going to fix things for them, but that I'm really there to have them express how they feel in movement. Because of that, they are able to be very open to me. There's no criticism, there's no expectation.

It is a mystery. You think that there's just red paint, blue paint, and yellow paint, but when you start mixing them together—wow!—you can get all these different shades and different colors. And that's what happens in healing art. You mix them, the three primary things, all together and the possibilities are endless. We do a lot of writing, poetic writing, where we just use single words and then try to put them together and then all these stories come out. Unbelievable. Energy is something you can see. You can't touch it, you can just call it part of that mystery. But there is something that doesn't make any logical sense that is happening in that room—impacting everybody. And it is going beyond the physical boundaries. It's some sort of energetic force, like a current in the environment. If you can't measure it and can't see it, it's like trying to imagine a color you've never seen.

Every part of the body speaks a different language; every part of the body has a particular song. If I'm working with the chest, it's very heartrending. It will bring up sadness, it will bring up joy. If I work with the feet, it will bring up grounding and strength and hanging on. If I work with the arms, it brings up reaching and drawing in. If I work with the spine, it brings out support. So I know that every part of the body has its own mythology, and within that mythology there's a basic emotion and image within that body part. So I can use that as a guide without imposing any personal judgments or any guessing. I can just plunge into the creative process right along with them. But there is that knowledge that if I'm going to work with the head, it's going to bring up the letting go of burdens, and if I'm going to use the hands to guide the head, I know that the hands are going to give that burden some compassion.

HOW TO HEAL YOURSELF WITH DANCE

STEP ONE: STARTING ON THE PATH
- Find a space to be your dance floor, where your movement can be free.
- Allow yourself to stretch to warm up.
- Connect with the energy inside your body.
- Allow your body to move spontaneously, and follow the movements.
- Select the music that you love or want to move to.
- Follow the rhythm of the music.

- Start to dance with explorations in pure movement.
- Allow the divine dancer to move within you.

STEP TWO: THE JOURNEY

- See each movement as a deliberate, conscious act.
- Make an intention to move in beauty and grace.
- Embody emotions as movements.
- Use your breath to create an ebb and flow.
- Use scarves to move air in flowing movements or to simulate water.
- Access your inner self through dance.
- Go to the place where emotion merges with movement.
- Allow sounds to emerge as you dance if that is natural.
- Be nonjudgmental; let go of criticism or expectation.
- Merge with the life force.

STEP THREE: DEEPENING

- Dance within the motions of your day.
- Draw images and then dance them.
- Dance symbols.
- Dance an animal.
- Dance a tree or rock.
- Dance an image or a feeling.
- Move to define space.
- Go deep inside your body.
- If you dance with others, make a lot of contact.
- Use imagery in your dance.
- Dance to connect with your soul.

STEP FOUR: TRANSCENDENCE

- Visualize your spirit and body becoming one.
- Feel yourself as a dance of pure light.
- Allow yourself to fall deeply into the center of a dancing spiral.
- Allow yourself to dance through life as you move.

- ◆ Receive the energy of the earth.
- ◆ Connect with the dancer in the stars.
- ◆ Honor the mystery of the dance.
- ◆ Create a sacred circle of witnesses to your dance.

Advice from Anna on Healing Yourself with Dance

My advice to a person who wants to heal herself with dance is to do whatever matches her calling. If she loves reading poetry, if that's something she loves to do, read the poem, then find a way to put that poem into a dance, memorize the poem and move as you're narrating the poem. If you love music, pick out ten different qualities of music—something based on a very soft sound, something very rhythmic, something very strong—and go to the store and get a selection of these different pieces of music. Play the music and just dance to the music—whatever the music says to you. Another thing is take a walk in nature and as you walk, touch, smell, feel, caress, hug. Do it by yourself or with a friend who is on the same path that you're on. Walk or, if you're in better condition, run.

I also advise everyone to draw. In the beginning, your drawings may seem like nothing, and you may think that you can't draw, but everybody can. I advise you to draw a body picture of yourself, and then you can do drawings of whatever images come up for you when you are moving. You can also do drawings of animals and things. At the end of every session, the second week before the end, I always have people find an animal ally through a meditation. I always have them draw it and dance it. It really is crucial to do the animal dance. Animals are totally spontaneous in terms of their responses to things. If a dog is happy, it wags its tail. Birds fly. We all have dreams of flying, so birds represent liberation and freedom. I always do animal allies, and they always have something important to say. You know we have four kinds of animals that we connect with movement: We have an animal under the ground, an animal on the ground, a hoofed animal, and an aerial animal. If people stay with me long enough, they get four animals of their own. I tell them they can also call on any of the animals. Animals are totally spontaneous with their feelings, and moving like them is another way for us to get at our own healing images. The other thing that is important is to identify with a stone and find that stillness, that unmovable strength of minerals. They can also identify with plants, finding their vertical growing energy.

TRANSCENDENCE IN DANCE

Jill Sonke Henderson tells us the story of a little girl with leukemia. Jill had been dancing with the little girl for weeks. She had been dancing with her each day. She danced the girl's fantasy of being in a fairy castle. Around this magic castle, both of them would dance to make the flowers grow. One day an evil witch came. She came to destroy everything. Jill and the little girl would make magic. They would dance together and by magic they would dance the flowers back. They would dance life back into the kingdom. Jill would play this out with the little girl every day. Under the little girl's direction she would dance out the little girl's dream. As they would dance they would tell stories. Each day the dance would change; each day it was new.

Then one day, the child told her mother that the bad cells were back. The doctors had all thought she was better but the little girl knew she wasn't. They found that a new tumor had grown quickly. When the little girl began to get sicker she said, "Mommy I am going to God, to the magical castle in the sky. I am going to dance with the angels and be free. Oh mommy, I love to dance."

One of the reasons we are writing this book is to understand this story. Art here is an embodied process that the child participates in. The process starts with the seemingly simple act of dancing in the room. Somewhere in the ordinary process of the dance, the child entered the spiritual realm of heaven. Within the dance she went into pure spirit and transcended her ordinary life. The dance was her way. The dancer was her helper to get there. The process was mysterious and staggeringly beautiful; it was transcendent in itself.

Healing dance somehow gives the little girl and the dancer a doorway where they can go from an embodied dance to a transcendental experience. They take the dance and go into themselves, into a place of transformation where they are free. Jill has said it takes them on the sacred spiral of art and healing. This is just Jill's way of trying to explain her personal experience of pure radiance. The magical process leads them to a place of love and to a place of transcendence at once.

In the dance, the creative act is simple. The dancer twirls her flowing scarf. The dancer's body enhances the possibilities of what the dance experience can be. In your mind's eye watch the dancer lift her arms, twirl, lift her legs, twirl, jump in the air, descend, seem to float. See the scarf sailing through the air, and see yourself in this ethereal, beautiful dancer as she gently twirls around the room. The dancer on the outside suddenly becomes the dancer within. You are the dancer.

NINE

HEALING YOURSELF WITH SOUND: MUSIC AS HEALING

This chapter is your invitation to use music as one of the most powerful healing modalities being rediscovered today. There is more research on music than on any other creative healing modality. It has been shown to alleviate stress, elevate moods, help with clear thinking, reduce pain, and promote healing. This is your opportunity to explore the ways you can introduce music into your life to facilitate your creative healing.

INTRODUCING YOUR MUSICIAN-IN-RESIDENCE

Pure excitement and joy come into your room with Dr. Peter Halprin. He says, "I will play you a song. Listen. I am a doctor who heals with music. This is what my whole life is about. It is where I have been. My name is Peter. I am a doctor, but I was a musician. I had to leave music to become a physician. For years, there was a time when I did medicine without music. Now, finally, I realize I can't do that anymore. Now I am a doctor who plays music with my patients. I play music to relax them, to help them remember who they are, to remind them of the past, to help them deal with emotions. Music is the most powerful healing force. Look, music has vibrations that

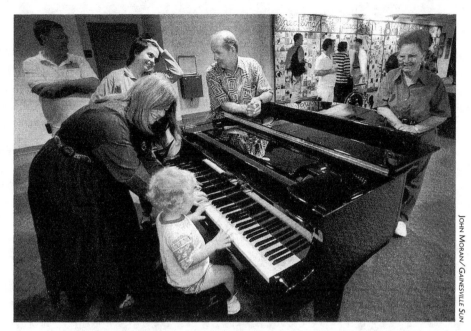

Cathy DeWitt Shows a Patient How to Play the Piano in the Hospital Atrium. Cathy is the musician-in-residence at Shands Hospital. Many musicians perform in hospitals across the country. This brings the spirit of music to the hearts of people who need healing. Music is going to be one of the most powerful tools of healing in the twenty-first century.

change every cell in your body. Music heals babies in hospitals. I have known that all my life, and now I can live it at last. This is the future of healing. Let me play you a song about healing. Close your eyes and listen."

As he plays his guitar, you can see Peter being himself at last, finding out who he is at last, bringing both sides of himself together at last. You can see his power rising, his spirit soaring, and his healer emerging. This physician is practicing the music healing of the future. This physician has awakened to the expanding and innovative possibilities of health care.

Peter Halprin is a physician who practices in Cape Cod, Massachusetts. He was a singer and guitarist before he went to medical school. Now, in addition to his medical practice, he lectures to caregivers on the value of healing music and performs his beautiful music in front of patients and caregivers to help them heal.

HOW SOUND HEALS

Sound creates vibrational shifts in the body. Sound is what our ears pick up from vibrations moving through air. There are actually air molecules moving in space. There is a motion with a rhythm and a frequency moving in space and time. Our bodies pick up the sound with our ears, and the rest of our body picks up the vibrations in every molecule of every cell. For example, sound brings the vibrations of your voice into your chest.

The voice is powerful; it can shift your whole emotional state from anger to love. You can use your voice to express love and healing intention. Sound is a way to create vibrational healing and bring love into your own body. You can use your voice as the vehicle for loving yourself. Any sound can be used—humming, chanting, singing, or repeating words to rhythm. Affirmations such as "I am one with my song" are very effective when put to a melody. You can use your voice to sing a lullaby to a baby or to sing child-hood songs to a very old person. Music transcends time; it brings us to places of feeling. It is the most physically accessible form of art. It is deeply embodied. It uses your own body as the vehicle for healing. The music is inside you, vibrating and changing the patterns of molecules in your cells. The snake uncoils in your body, singing to the bones, singing from your heart.

Ancient healers used chanting and singing to evoke the spirit. They called to the spirits in chants, stories, and song. We praise God and evoke our lovers with music. We use song to relax, feel ecstasy, raise our energy, and have fun. We listen to gospel songs to elevate our soul, love songs to put us in the mood for love. Music affects our mood instantly; it uplifts, lowers; it can facilitate emotional energy shifts powerfully and quickly. We can use music as a tool to effect change. We can use it with intent to heal and relax.

Anyone can use chanting with the intent of making music to heal. We can chant into our bodies. We can sing to one another. We can sing to our grandmothers; we can sing to them of their childhood, and they will get up and become young again. Music can take people into a timeless place, where they can be somewhere else again. It can take them to an ancient past. It can take them into the place where they know God. How fast do you feel joy and open your heart when you hear certain songs on the radio? You go from being depressed to being as happy as you can be in one moment. You don't do anything, you are taken there by the music.

Music is going to be one of the most powerful tools of healing in the twenty-first century. There is much literature to validate and support this belief. The practice of music healing has not caught up to the research and does not reflect the enormous amount of literature that proves the richness of this medium in healing. This medium has already been applied successfully in nursing homes, hospitals, intensive-care units, and even people's own homes. Creative ways of applying the medium will be part of the future of healing.

BECOMING ONE WITH TONES

Edie Hartshorne is a therapist who uses music to heal. A woman she worked with was having problems in her marriage and felt alienated from her husband. Edie worked with her to choose sounds and tones that made her feel at one with herself. First the woman picked her instruments. She chose Tibetan bowls of different sizes and tones. She would simply play them and meditate and listen to the sounds. She would close her eyes and daydream as the tones went though her body. Next she put the bowls on her body and toned the sounds that seemed to make her feel most at peace. She then thought of doing this with her husband, and he spent time with her as she played her bowls. The tones carried them away in a meditative state that brought them closer together and made them feel at one with each other. As her music deepened, so did their relationship. She felt she knew herself intimately as she went into her tones, and as she knew who she was, she let herself love her husband for who he was. Art and healing is the most basic mind-body therapy.

Edie's Advice on How to Use Music to Heal Yourself

I suggest that people get a tape. You can use all sorts of music. Now there is a whole genre of healing music. There is also music that is done live, that is acoustical, that has only pure sounds. There are some tapes of Tibetan bells, and the tapes I make have flutes and bells.

When my son died, I could not listen to anything except *Rosa Mystica*, played by Terese Shreder Shaker. I think that people know what is healing for them. I suggest that people listen to music with nothing else going on. Lie down on a sofa or a bed for ten minutes, not much more than that, put the music on, turn the phones off. Say, "This is the time that I am healing my body." Say, "I am giving my dear body attentive, faithful healing." It is amazing how refreshing that can be. And I suggest that it be music that is quite slow, and that you breathe with the music. The music that we record is all done with breath, so it is extremely easy to breathe with it. You begin to feel the beat of the music, and in that way your heart slows down, your breath goes into your belly, and you feel refreshed. It is cheap, easy, quick. Anybody can do it, any time, any place.

Playing music yourself is not necessary. But I also believe that anybody can play music, and that you can start at any age. I think that it is a wonderful thing to begin to play an instrument as an older person. And from my experience of starting to play Japanese music in my middle forties, I found that you have to have "beginners' mind."

Japanese music is not at all like Western music. When I started, it was like I was a baby. I thought, "A cute little five-year-old could play this music that I can't." It is a fabulous way to experience what it is really like to start learning like a child. You can experience what it is like to really start from the beginning, and you realize how absurd it is that we criticize ourselves. So it is a fabulous experience in self-awareness. And if you do it without becoming attached to the idea of being a great performer but rather to just see what this experience is like, then you can enjoy the simplest tune. You just play a few notes and experience what it is like to make the sound. And there are people you can find who will teach you in this way. You can buy movable xylophones, where you strike the bells that sound gorgeous, and if you set it up in a pentatonic scale, it is beautiful. You can't make any mistakes. You can buy a little harp that is pentatonic. I have done this with two-

or three-year-olds and with adults. They take a single note, and I say to them, "That is your note," and the person sings only that note. You can really become as interested in one single note as you can in a whole piece.

There are lots of ways that people can experience music as an adult. And, of course, the human voice is wonderful. You can tone and chant with a little bell so that you are accompanying yourself. Start in the shower. You can also begin to match the sounds that you hear in the environment. For example, when a train goes by, it makes a certain pitch. You can listen to that sound and you can slide your voice so that you match it. You feel it in your body. In that moment, you are entrained. You can use this when there is an annoying sound. When you match the sound, it does not bother you. You can do this with every sound. If you turn on the hair dryer, it gives a note. If you are with a friend and you put the dryer on low and then high, each sound is a note you can tone together. Toning in the bathroom is great. If you turn on the shower, you won't feel as embarrassed. It is very good for your body and it feels great.

You can also learn sacred chants. I chant the Buddhist lovingkindness meditation every morning with my husband. I start first myself, then we say the names of anyone who needs prayer, and we chant that person's name, and at the end of the five minutes of chanting we feel refreshed. It is a different way of saying a prayer. Whenever someone is in need or ill or in danger, we chant their name. And people will call us to do it for them.

I want to say something about the music of nature. I experience the sounds of nature to be as powerful as music, especially if I am away from the freeway or electricity. When I come back to the city, my body vibrates in a higher frequency, so I think that for me what is almost more powerful than music is the silence in the sound of the wind. The wind in the cottonwood trees is different. Different trees have a different sound. I love no sound or the sound of fog. There is a quality of sound in fog that enwraps you. I was in fog in a rain forest three years after my son died and I felt an incredible intensity. I was very hot. I heard a voice, and I felt his presence all around me. In the fog I heard, "Haven't you noticed I have been here all the time? I have been with you always." And that moment was the moment when I was able to begin to heal.

I think music was the golden thread that led me back to my true self. Listen, listen—this wonderful sound takes me back to my true self. And that is what made the difference. For years and years I had no voice. When I was growing up, I could barely speak in class. I would shake. I could never say what I meant. I had these powerful feelings that felt so incoherent. I was a child of the fifties; I grew up "standing behind the man." I looked extroverted, but it wasn't until I started playing Japanese music that I was freed. The virulent superego critics were not so noisy, and then I began to come out of myself. I came to the music as a way to find myself, to find my voice.

And having been through the journey myself, I know what it is like to feel that I have something to say, but not to know how. I know how you feel inside when you know you have the jewel and you don't know how to express it. I want to open the way so everyone can experience what it is like when you allow the jewel to be seen. It takes study and craft to give the jewel its shape, but study of an art is simple when you do it each day. You do it. It is nothing magical. People separate making art from themselves. That is a split that is totally wrong. Everyone who can sing, can make art. We split our creativity, and people feel they can't do it. They identify artists as people other than themselves. That is a great inner sadness, because it is our nature to want to reveal this beauty that we all experience. And it is in the nature of the human species to want to share that. It is our nature to create art and to witness creative healing. That is why it is as if you are listening to the divine in me, and you let me know it. The one who listens is giving the artist the great gift. As a musician, how can I not be ecstatic when someone says, "I see the divine joy coming from you"? It is a wonderful experience everyone should have. We witness one another; we encourage one another to speak.

HOW TO HEAL YOURSELF WITH MUSIC

STEP ONE: STARTING ON THE PATH

- Find a time each day and listen to music consistently.
- Pick tapes that you love that resonate with you.
- Close your eyes and listen.
- Turn the phones off.
- Let music take you elsewhere.
- Breathe with the music.
- Get in touch with each sound.
- Return to the pleasure of music.
- Find a place to sing, tone, or chant.
- Experience the sounds of nature.

STEP TWO: THE JOURNEY

- Make music an intentional part of healing.
- Play music to relax.
- Listen to tapes of music that are healing.
- Bring tapes to any stressful event or medical procedure.
- Make your own tape library.
- Say no to hostile or jarring sounds.
- Listen to sounds that balance you.
- Become one with the sound.
- Feel the rhythm in your body.
- Hum or chant.
- Sing or repeat words to a rhythm.
- Sing in the shower.
- Tone in the shower.
- Try playing an instrument like a child, with joy and without judgment.
- Take up a new instrument.
- Walk along a stream or brook and listen.
- Go to the music of the ocean, a brook, or a waterfall and listen.
- Listen to the wind, to fog.

- Listen to birds.
- Feel the harmony of the sound surround you.

STEP THREE: DEEPENING
- Feel the power rise within you.
- Allow the vibrational shifts in your body to move through you.
- Repeat affirmations such as "I am one with my song" to music.
- Sing a lullaby to yourself or a loved one.
- Invite friends to serenade you with music.
- Have a friend play the guitar and sing to you.
- Make your own instrument with things that are around.
- Use repetitive sound rhythms as an inner chant.

STEP FOUR: TRANSCENDENCE
- Imagine your spirit soaring as song.
- Sing to your bones.
- Sing from your heart.
- Evoke your God with music and song.
- Learn sacred chants.
- Listen to silence.
- Put yourself in the center of a healing circle of music.
- Make a drumming circle for healing.
- Listen to the earth's body sing to you.
- Turn up the volume of nature's healing music.
- Create a community of music makers.
- Form singing circles.

MUSIC HEALS IN AN INSTANT

Music simply can change a situation immediately. Picture a room in a bone marrow transplant ward. It is arid; nothing is there to raise your spirits. There are machines, pumps, tubes. The child is lying there so sick he does not even move. His eyes are fixed and half open in pain and in fear. The experience is a lot more than you can bear. The child is sick and tired of suffering; his mother is there almost on the edge of collapse. All of a sudden, a young man with a guitar comes in. He shuffles in awkwardly. He is uncomfortable at first. It is a strange surrounding. His guitar is on his back, and he is always uncomfortable in these kinds of hospital rooms. He wants to say something. The child looks at the young man, not sure of what he wants. He looks like he will make a request. Then the young man offers to play the child a song.

Suddenly, the man's awkwardness transforms into joy. He transforms into the musician that he is. He brings out his guitar from the case. "Hi, my name is Dan, I am a musician, and I work in the hospital program." Suddenly his energy shifts. He is exuberant. The child is still not sure what he means. "I don't want a song," the child says. The young man says, "I'll play you a song. What is your favorite song? I think I know that." He sits on the edge of the bed. He holds his guitar and sings the song. Suddenly there is a smile. The child is too weak to sing, but he smiles gently. The young man sings to the child every day, serenading him as he goes deep into his dreams.

In another moment, a mother is with a baby who is screaming. The baby cries, arches his back. Everyone is having a hard time. The mother pats him on the back; the baby is so difficult. He is so uncomfortable he is in pain. The mother sits down in a rocking chair and sings the baby a lullaby. She begins to hum from her belly. She feels the sound, the vibrations from her chest. The baby is still crying. She feels the energy rising in her, her love rising in her chest with the sound. The baby starts to whimper instead of cry. The mother sways back and forth like a dancer, singing a sweet lullaby as ancient as the stars. The baby quiets; he looks up at her so softly. He drifts off to sleep; he is calm and suddenly peaceful. This is how music heals. Feel the beauty of the moment, feel the ancient piety of the moment. That is how music heals.

The Recycled Trash Queens were formed by a group of women who were drummers. They came into the hospital and used recycled trash to make music. They used all kinds of cans, milk cartons, orange juice containers, anything that was trash and could make a sound. In the hospital, they would put all the trash on a table. Then the kids would make drums. They took pots and pans and anything that would make a sound. The kids would start drumming. The women were drummers, after all, so they could make drumming sounds from anything. You can be as creative and have as much fun as this. This was a simple project that brought music into a pediatric ward in a large hospital. It worked. It was easy and effective. They would put on concerts in the atrium with recycled trash and have everyone play. It demystified the music making of healing music. It showed that healing music can be done by anyone with anything. The diversity and variety of musicians—from drummers to guitar players—capture the imagination as the minstrels of the old world did. These wandering musicians bring in songs and stories from another world and travel into these places of darkness where healing light must occur.

Lewis Played Guitar for Nancy as She Died

Michael tell us this story of his younger son, Lewis:

> When my wife, Nancy, was dying of breast cancer, our younger son, Lewis, would serenade her for hours. She was in a liver coma from liver metastasis and was starting to lose consciousness. It was slow and gentle but totally real. Lewis was sixteen years old, and Nancy had been sick since he was twelve. One month before, the metastasis in her liver and lungs had grown rapidly. Her two physicians had set up a special meeting to tell her. They met in an office across from the hospital, so neither would be alone with this woman whom they had learned to love over the four years they had taken care of her. When she heard the news she did not cry. She looked right at them, and her only reaction was to ask if she could still go to England to visit English gardens. She had planned the trip for the whole spring, and it was one thing she looked forward to deeply. I could see them both roll their eyes and look away, and then her medical oncologist, Sam Spivak, paused. "Of course you can, Nancy," he said, so gently. Later I heard that he told a friend that if he were to die, he would just as soon die in an English garden. But she not only survived the trip; she almost was not impaired on it. She ran through the gardens, sometimes two or three a day, her bald head covered with a hat, a raincoat protecting her from the damp English spring, her face radiant and at peace. In

a strange way, she was deeply at home. Her spirit was free. Once I saw her sitting on a bench at the end of a long path of hedges. You could see the light around her rising. It was so beautiful.

When she returned home, her body rapidly became more ill. Her liver function tests were very high, and she started to fall asleep and wake up alternately. As usual, she did not want to know how long she had to live, but she wanted to make plans so her children could be with her. She did not want Rudy, our older son, to travel from home as he was planning, so she asked me to call Sam, her oncologist, and ask him if Rudy could go on a trip. The night before she had told me that her relationship with Lewis needed to be healed for her. He was a teenager and she had had trouble talking closely to him as she was dying, and now she needed some resolution without discussing death. Lewis was in the living room when I called Sam. He understood what I was asking Sam and why. He had been through this kind of call before. On the phone, Sam told me that Rudy should not leave even for a week. I hung up and told Nancy that Sam had said that Rudy could not travel. Tears came to her eyes, which was exceedingly rare. She paused, and Lewis came up to her and kissed her and said, "I love you, mother." That was unusual for him, too. I could see her body loosen up and open and her spirit rise. It was as if a weight had been taken off of her. She had her resolution.

The next day she went upstairs into our loft overlooking the ocean and the mountains, never to come down again alive. She went into our bed where both boys had been conceived, nursed with love, and read to and sung to as babies and started to hold a sacred beingness. Rachel Remen, in her book *Kitchen Table Wisdom,* called Nancy's state before her death "sitting Dashan," the state where a guru gives gifts to her followers. When Nancy's best friend, Elizabeth, came, she said that Nancy had turned into pure love. She had. Her personality had departed and in its place was her eternal soul. She would only say to each person who visited her, "I love you so much, you are so beautiful, I am so happy to see you." She gave each person the gift of love as they came to pay their last respects and say good-bye.

Meanwhile, Lewis and Rudy, both her boys, made healing art, each in his own way. Rudy dug an enormous fish pond next to Nancy's English garden. He made her "garden art." It took his whole body and all his physical energy. It was digging in the earth; it was like a huge grave. He would dig and come upstairs and sit and tell stories and go down and dig when she was asleep. Lewis had his own rhythm. He would go downtown and surf and then would come home and sit next to her bed whether she was asleep or awake and play his guitar. He was writing a soft, slow piece for her death that was so beautiful. I think it came right from his heart or from somewhere else far deeper. He would work on the song and play to her throughout the days as she looked at him, as she had visitors, as she slept in her coma, as she dreamed. His guitar piece grew and was like an endless round. It circled and caressed you like the wind. It came around your body like her love and carried you and made you feel taken care of, blessed, and in the hands of a greater force. He just sat and played it for hours; it seemed endless. It was acoustic guitar, soft and caring. And as she dreamed, she drifted with him, and he carried her. She floated on the music, and he cared for her perfectly in her last days on earth as his mother.

THE SOUNDS OF NATURE HEAL

There is healing music in the natural sounds of the earth. There is healing in the sound of the gentle wind, in the sound of the stream, in the sound of the ocean. There is healing in the owl's call, in the sound of the waves, in the sound of the waterfall. Go to the music of the ocean, and listen to the sound of the natural world. Sit on the edge of a brook next to a waterfall, and go to the place where you can hear the music of the earth's body. This sound is what we hear. It is the sound of the air, water, fire, and earth moving. It is what we hear in the vibrations going deep into every cell in our body. These are great places of healing energy. The energy vibrates and shifts into patterns and changes us. By just being inside the sound you can soothe your body. These sounds are the earth's songs. She is singing to you. This is part of healing music. And listening to the changes of the earth's body as she moves is healing. Listen to the change as she moves in storms; listen to the change as she moves in thunder, in the strong wind blowing. These are all musical songs of the earth. They are faded in our culture. They are dimmed by television and even radio. The earth herself will heal you with sound. Places that still have the sounds of the earth are places on our planet that are greatly healing. Listen to the earth's body dance as a healing song. Sit on the edge of a stream that comes from a redwood forest and hear the earth sing to you and tell you that she loves you.

As you sit by a waterfall on the rocks, know that she has brought you to a mountain stream and put you in the center of her song. She wanted you to hear her sound. "This is the sound of the earth's body," she said. "You could listen to it forever. Move to a bigger waterfall; that will turn up the volume." We walk past this kind of sound every day and don't realize that this is music healing.

Turn up the volume on nature's healing music in your life. Healing with music is going to the ocean every week. These natural sounds are the music of the earth. You can listen to them on tape in a hospital room, but they are even more wonderful to listen to in nature. Go to these sounds with the intention of balancing yourself, and become one with the sound. Allow the sound to go into your body. Feel the harmony of the sound. Let it go into your body to where you need it.

SINGING TO OTHERS AS HEALING

Singing to heal can be as simple as making up songs, for yourself if you are ill, for your children if they are sick, or for your loved ones if they need you. Or it can be bringing music to Alzheimer's patients, singing them songs from their childhood. For them, the music resonates, sparking the embodied memories of the time they were lucid and free. Often just singing a familiar song for Alzheimer's patients makes them completely lucid for a moment, and they can sing along and be happy. This is a perfect example of the healing power of sound in music. You do it, and you can see it is powerful.

Just singing brings a person out of a demented state and makes them animated and engaged and feel young again.

Music and healing is the most researched area of art and healing. There are more studies of music and healing than of any other art form. There are hundreds of studies of music as a health-care intervention (see the bibliography). There are studies of music and pain relief, music and attitude, music and relaxation. The question now is, How can we implement music in patient care? Why is it not a reality in each of our lives when we are ill? How can it be used in the hospital room, at home, in nursing homes? The easiest way is through CDs and cassette tapes and through singing to one another. It is especially important to bring music to children who are ill. And bringing music back into institutions such as hospitals and schools that are not healthy in themselves is crucial. Healing music needs to be in our environment. Open the windows to hear natural sounds. Protect the resources of natural healing sounds, like trees and streams, around us.

Michael tells this story:

> One time I was at Esalen teaching a workshop. I had a massage and the woman who did it sang to me. She picked me up as she did the massage and gently rocked me in her arms. She sang a song that sounded like a lullaby, it was so soft and caring. I was amazed. I closed my eyes and drifted off with the music; I opened my eyes and looked at her above me rocking me. It was so primal. It obviously brought me back to the times I had been rocked and sung to by my mother when I was a little baby. Music is deeply healing, in the most primal ways. Using it with healing intent combined with massage is very powerful.

THE COMMUNITY OF MAKING MUSIC

It is extremely valuable to join with others in a community making music with the intent to heal. If you are ill, put yourself in the center of a circle of chanting or singing. In Western medicine, we are just beginning to find out how sound can be used in group healing experiences, and how the sound of others making music with intent to heal can be used best. Healing musicians make music to heal with people who are ill. Feel the vibrations pulsate in your own body.

We can form singing circles from our own community. We can bring people together who will sing and make music with intent to heal. Make a singing circle in your living room; bring it to a sick child's hospital bed. Bring a singing circle to a nursing home. Bring a singing circle to your aging parents. This is a way we can come together. It is a way that is very ancient, a way that we as humans have always used to touch one another's souls.

Vicki Noble is a woman healer who uses music, chanting, and drumming in large group healing circles. Her work in music healing is innovative and groundbreaking. She works with individuals with many illnesses, including brain tumors and cancers of all kinds. It is a primal ancient healing practice. In her work, she gets together at least thirty and as many as one hundred women to form an intentional group healing circle. She also uses a community circle of drummers to keep a rhythm. The drumming maintains a rhythm that is constant and takes people deeper and deeper into their bodies. She has the singers sing a simple chant, such as "Purify us and heal us; heal us and free us." Everyone sings the chant with the drumming. The people who need to be healed are put in the center of the circle. The chanters chant until all thoughts and even all words are gone. Everyone then can be totally focused on healing. They then employ the technique of laying on of hands.

Vicki believes that her technique uses the body of the earth to heal. She believes it takes going into the rhythm of the earth to change the rhythm of an illness. As the rhythm changes, the person who is ill opens up to the energies of the earth and to the other healers. The process is very physical, and Vicki believes that energetically it takes at least an hour of chanting to make the breakthrough. She believes that the fire of the earth in your own body comes out. Huge circles of intentional healing are intense and powerful. We believe that this kind of work is futuristic and creative and exciting. It challenges us to create innovative ways to use music and art to heal. Presently, Vicki is attempting to do research to demonstrate that her group music healing can cure cancer. She has anecdotal evidence that patients have had remissions from cancer after her process. The point is that everyone is an artist. Everyone can do this kind of work. You are a healer and an artist. You can heal yourself by just bringing out the artist that you are. This work is simple and can be done by anyone.

TONING AND SOUND AS VIBRATION

Music and sound have a vibratory quality that actually changes the physical body. One way of looking at sound healing is that vibration affects the molecules and cells in the body. The vibration itself causes the body's fluid and particles to move and rearrange. This way of looking at sound is new for medical science but as ancient as healing. Sound healers have always believed that vibration changed the body structure. Sacred music healing was always based on the sacred music having pure and ancient vibrations that would make people heal by putting them into perfect harmony.

In this way of looking at music, it is the vibrational energy that actually changes physiology. Sound waves set up patterns in matter. The complexity of the sound vibrations are observable and have been demonstrated in research films. The human body as a vibrational form is always moving toward regeneration and increasing complexity. The sound vibrations break up blockages and set up new patterns. With cancer, you use the sound to create harmony and balance. You use it as a conduit to find the place inside you that has innate wisdom. You use sound vibration to dislodge any rigid pattern that has formed and needs to be transformed into something to be healed. In this model, illness is seen as a dysfunctional pattern. Music is a way to deal with shifting rhythms of the body on a cellular level.

Sound healing has always been done along with intent, prayer, and affirmations. It is a type of inner transpersonal imagery healing that uses a sound instead of a visual image. What is important here is the inner chanting. Repeating the rosary is an example of this type of healing. You use the inner chant and sound rhythm to get into the place of healing. Prayer, mantras, and affirmations are all vehicles to put yourself in the healing state, where your intent can come out unfettered. Inner chanting is a simple way to use sound in a repetitive method that takes you out of thought and emotion and puts you deep into your body. It creates a sound pattern that is removed from thought.

It places the individual into a spatial vibrating form of their own consciousness or into a place of oneness with God or spirit. It is like reuniting with the
sound of your own heartbeat or breathing. You are returning to the source of
life by going into its pure sound. You are returning to the place where the life
force is strongest. Sound has always been combined with the rhythm of prayer
and the power of word. This kind of healing can be used in every culture. It is
understood and can be learned in every language. It is as ancient in its origins
as any spiritual practice or belief. We need to return to it. Its simplicity makes
it an easy way for any of us to heal ourselves or others with music.

SILENCE AS SOUND HEALING

Inside sound there is also an experience of silence. Silence is the sound of
no sound. It is the purest form of sound. You are listening with your ears as
acutely as you listen to music, but no sound is heard. Silence is the pause
between beats, the space between vibrations. Silence is no vibration. Silence
is something we can cultivate in our lives. This is essential in a time when
you are working on your own personal healing. There are many strategies to
cultivating the spaciousness of silence. Different types of meditation focus
your attention on your breath. Even if you don't have a time commitment to
do this, you can go into the place of silence within yourself. Even in the
busy moments of your life, within a moment you can find the silence that is
eternally spacious, that can connect you to your own soul.

There are moments in your life when you can remember the experience
of silence. In silence, there is a fullness and spaciousness of being intensely
alive. It is being truly present. In the silence, you find your deepest wisdom
and greatest sense of being in your body. In the silence, you can see the richness of how life is alive, vibrant, and colorful. In the moment of slipping into
the silence, it is as if you have opened the spaces between the breaths. It is
like going inside the moments. It is a way of getting in between the moments
of time. This can be as simple as going into the woods and taking a walk and
listening to the silence. And as simple as being with the fullness of the
silence inside yourself. In silence is a place of peace, of stillness, and of com-
pletion. In silence, you are perfect the way you are.

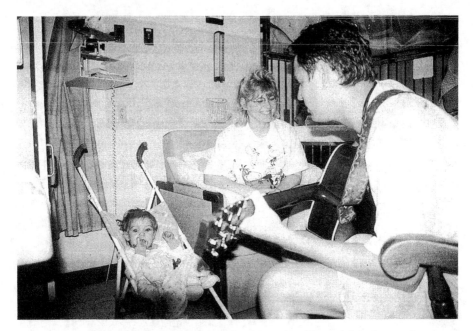

The Strolling Musician Serenades Us. Dan plays his guitar and sings a lullaby for a mother and her baby. The simple act of his coming into the room and singing songs is one of the most beautiful art and healing forms.

Within the striving to get well, there is an experience of already being well. Inside of you is a place of balance already. You can get there with the silence. Allow your thoughts to flow. Let them go. Cultivate the experience of allowing yourself to be in a flow. It can be as simple as focusing on the breath. Go deeper into the inner world of silence or into the pause. It may be about being with God, or one with love. It is about emerging out of the experience of compassion.

There are silences inside each and every art form. It is the pause in any process. The pause before your next breath, where nothing is moving and there is only the life force manifest as desire. It is within the fluidity of movement. It is within the flow that is natural. When you are in pain, stress, or conflict, fall into silence and don't feel that you have to do anything. It is music healing without music.

THE STROLLING MUSICIAN AS A HEALER

As an artist-in-residence, the musician is sometimes like a gypsy artist, a wanderer. His name is Dan, and one day he was asked to see a young girl. She was sixteen and very sick. She was close to his age, just a teenager. She was unresponsive at first, very bloated, and slipping into a coma. The staff would just sit with her and did not know what to do to help her. The musician went into her dark room, where the shades were drawn. It was a room filled with sadness. He asked her if she would like a song to be sung to her. She was much too sick to even speak back to him, but she looked up with her eyes. He chose "Brown-Eyed Girl." He sang the song to her softly; he sat on her bed, and as he played, tears ran down her face. She could not speak, but she mouthed the words. The art reached her on a level that was so deep, it connected her with a precious moment in her past of just living. Deep in the process of her illness she went far below her thoughts. Music created a palpable full emotional experience. There is nothing more beautiful than being serenaded at the foot of a bed. We take it for granted in the ways that it can connect people, but it is more powerful than anything else we have. The event was a little miracle filled with life and love.

The strolling musician has always been a romantic image. In our dreams, it was always just a handsome young man who played a guitar, serenading his lover under a window. The musician-in-residence at Shands Hospital would go from room to room serenading each patient. He would serenade young girls who were very ill, mothers and babies after delivery, old people who were alone. The simple act of his coming into the room and singing songs is the most beautiful art and healing form. It was, after all, as simple as a musician or lover coming in with his sensitivity and care. He is bringing love into each person's room. These young guitarists are among the most powerful healing artists. We invite everyone who can play the guitar and sing to come into patients' rooms and serenade them. It is a romantic image of the young man with the guitar that can come alive again. Honor this obscure musician. Like a strolling minstrel, he is unattached; he is filled with incredible beauty. We can't have a world without him. We are asking him to return.

LISTENING TO MUSIC TO HEAL YOURSELF

Tapes of favorite music are deeply healing for anyone who is facing illness or medical procedures. A cancer patient can play music while having procedures done and while waiting. Playing tapes in the hospital room changes the whole room and the patient's whole experience of being ill. The cassette player or CD player is a basic healing tool and a necessity for anyone who is ill or in a hospital. We believe that no one should go into a hospital without a way to listen to their favorite music. Many hospitals have cassette players available to patients who do not have their own. The boombox-type players are now so inexpensive that they are wonderful gifts for anyone who is ill and does not have one. Buy one instead of flowers for someone you are going to visit. Bring them your favorite healing music, whether it be the theme from *Chariots of Fire* or a Gregorian chant.

Any tape you love is what is right. Pick any tape that resonates with you. Go with your favorite music, whether it is jazz, classical, or popular. Pick anything that puts you in a mood that will center you and balance you in your life. You are striving for harmony. You need to start to respond to your body's rhythms. Remember, music can change your emotions to anything, so choose where you want to go. You can use it to meditate, to be calm and serene. You can use it to get energized, brave, confident, powerful. Find a time in your day that you use it consistently. You can do it more easily if there is consistency. You can use music to move you toward happiness if you are depressed. Use music as a tool in your life to evoke change in the moment. Music is a tool that is accessible to you all the time. Make choices that are healthy. Have confidence in your choices. Use music to center you when you exercise, cook dinner, drive your car. Make choices about the sound and song of what you put into your body. If you are sick, turn off anything hostile and abusive. Say no to those sounds. Say no to anything in the world that will make you sicker. The sounds go into your body on a vibrational level. They go into your consciousness and can be harmful. You know what they are. Listen to sounds that make you feel healthy and healing.

What makes someone happy, energized, relaxed, and spiritually uplifted is different for each person. A teenager has a completely different way of reacting to music than an adult or a child. Obviously, loud, fast music does not relax most people, but it may relax a teenager used to doing homework to this kind of sound. Recordings of relaxation instructions combined with music are also valuable. You can make your own recordings of friends or loved ones wishing you well or just speaking to you. You can record your family sitting around the dinner table with music in the background. So make your own list of music for the types of healing you need. Put together a tape or CD library that is relaxing, sleep inducing, energizing, uplifting, humorous, prayerful, memory evoking. You can use tapes during dental work and outpatient surgery or in situations that could be uncomfortable. They distract your attention and relax you and diminish pain and anxiety.

Michael's wife, Nancy, mastered the use of music to help her deal with breast cancer. She would use cassette tapes to deal with procedures, scans, surgery, getting news, relaxation, and going to sleep. She would go to concerts to raise her spirits when things were very bad. Whenever she had a procedure, whether a bone marrow aspiration or a scan, she would bring her Walkman and extra batteries. She would carry two or three tapes with her and decide which to play when she was there and felt the energy. If she needed relaxation, she would play Don Campbell's bells; if she needed joy she would play Van Morrison; if she needed uplifting she would play her chants. Now, this was not thought out rationally; it was just felt and done. No words or labels were put on the process, not even "healing with music"; it was just the natural thing to do. It worked. She used her tapes to go into surgery, come out in the recovery room, and recover in her hospital room. In her hospital room and in her bedroom at home, she had a cassette player that played the tapes out loud. She had a whole tape library of healing music that she had bought and that friends had given her as gifts. Friends would bring her music they loved, they would put together tapes of all their favorite pieces, they would give her spoken word prayers and chants. In her hospital room, she would play music twenty-four hours a day. Friends and nurses would ask her what she wanted to hear and would change the tapes for her all night if she was awake.

Michael tells this story:

On the day Nancy got the news that her breast cancer had metastasized to her lungs, she decided to go to a Van Morrison concert. It was difficult—it was in an inaccessible area of the city, parking was hard; it was like a pilgrimage. When you get the first news of the spread of breast cancer, it is very upsetting. This is the big news you don't want to get; it changes your life. It is deeply shocking and destabilizing and depressing. It is something huge to deal with. We sat in the back row of the large concert hall and listened to the loud music. She wanted to be alone and there at once. Van Morrison was far away; he looked as small as a play figure our children had had as babies. He was lit up in the brightest light. He was dancing, moving, jumping, opening up. He was singing her favorite songs, songs she had listened to after surgery and as she recovered at home, songs she had listened to as she dealt with her first diagnosis and as she put her life back together in her garden. She closed her eyes and flew with the music. She was so happy there. I could see her dropping into herself and becoming at home, and actually restructuring her worldview. I was in tears and barely holding it together. She was concentrating on the music in the moment, completely involved, elsewhere, in the place where music comes from in her heart. She was in her place of joy, healing, and being able to be fully alive even in this time. This music was her cue, her vehicle, and she knew it, and that is why we were there.

Making songs as the stories of our lives, with rhythm and momentum, is deeply healing. To do this, you make up your own songs and play music with them. We need to gather up the invaluable resource of musicians into our ordinary lives to make healing music. The time has come to look at the musician as a living person, not only as a stage reality. It transcends the concept of music as only for performance. Building bridges of music that is more personal will let everyone make music again. There are musicians who sing in church or school choruses. If we can extend this valuable resource into hospitals, into retirement homes, into people's lives, music can return to the world. If you are a musician, simply sing to the world. The world needs you now.

PART 3

HOW PROFESSIONAL ARTISTS ARE USING ART TO HEAL

TEN

THE WELLSPRING: HOW TO BECOME A HEALING ARTIST, AN ARTIST HEALER

We invite you to become a healing artist. As a healing artist, you become renewed. You have a chance to live your life over again. In your rebirth, you have gone through the fire and have emerged. It can take days, months, or years. It can take your whole life to learn how to express yourself in your creative work. It is about listening to the voice of the earth to heal; it is about listening to the voice of the earth to heal her.

As you change, you go to a place where you are the one who has wisdom, who is steadied by experience and has something important to share with others. Even if you have not been making healing art for long, your previous creative experiences give you something to share with others. Who you are in your creative form is the person the world needs. The healing artist says to you in the depth of your despair, "You can do this. I see the artist in there. I know you are creative. I can see you will get to the other side. It is right, it is your path. You will grow and you will change." That is what you have to share; it is your knowledge of this voice.

HEALING ARTISTS HONOR THE PEOPLE THEY WORK WITH

As a healing artist, you have to be committed to being an advocate for another person's freedom of self-expression and autonomy. Support another person's vision. You can become part of another person's life. You become part of their illness experience, part of their grief, their place, even their room. You help them experience their own world in a more creative way. You support their desire to be honored and served in the moment. It is simply about being truly present. It is simply about art as a way of caring. We care by going deeper into the other individual's desire for freedom, life, and self-expression. Patients as artists own their own art; they are free in their expression. You can engage them and make art with them. You can help them express themselves without any judgment or criticism. They can then tap into their own healer.

Healing artists must provide the leadership and commitment to integrate the arts into the healing models that exist in our culture today. The healing artist is in a unique position to offer partnerships between artists and healers to incorporate the arts into care. Art offers us a new way of seeing and being. The healing artist crystallizes the beauty that is always present, seeing the moment as it occurs, recognizing each healing encounter as important. It is a way of seeing, a way of making the invisible visible, hearing the unsung song, and listening to the untold stories. We are artists holding hands, listening to spirit. In this new partnership, art is a way of caring.

CHANGING THE WORLD OF ART

Some artists find that when they become studio artists and are involved in the art world, it is not enough. What is available to you as an artist in the art world may be too restrictive. The traditional art world is about galleries, exhibitions, openings, agents, museums, selling art, promotion. That life is about art that is collected and sold. It is frustrating for many artists today. They feel alone; their life is difficult and limited in its social interactions to "Will you buy my paintings?" "What was the review?" Many artists find that this is not the lifework for them. So there needs to be a way as a healing artist, or an artist healer, to change this. Healing art creates meaningfulness, richness, and environmental beauty.

Art is a spiritual path, but to actualize that vision, the artist needs to go out and recreate meaning. So for the healing artist, there is a mission to change the world of art. There is more to art than the art gallery. Art belongs in everyone's life. Like Susie Gablik, in her book *The Reenchantment of Art,* we ask artists to move out of their studios and into the community, into hospitals, businesses, and schools. But you have to do this yourself. You cannot expect the world to come to you and get you and tell you it needs art. Healing art is an activist movement. We are asking you to go into the hospitals and the schools as artists, so the world informs your work. Stop living in isolation. Healing art is about responsibility and responsiveness. Being a healing artist in our culture means being a facilitator to make art accessible to everyone. Just making your art accessible does that.

A CALL TO ARTISTS

The world needs you as a healing artist. You can go into patients' rooms when they are very ill, and you will be awed by the difference you will make in their day. You need to do this. This is what the world needs now to be healed. The healing wall of tiles at Shands Hospital in Gainesville, Florida, is a small glimmer of what is possible. The artists thought that they were only making tiles with patients and families. They almost didn't know why they were there. It turned out to be a memorial, reflecting the precious moments in the lives of the people who made the tiles. A man with lung cancer put his son's hand on his own and painted them as one. He looked deeply into his boy's eyes and saw him and his flow of generations, and the little hand within the big one made him cry. The artist shared in this moment. Each tile was a moment of illumination; each was so much more than the artist imagined. You can do this kind of healing, even if it is only one time in your life. This chapter is a call to artists. What is your vision? What is your dream? If you could do anything you wanted to, without failing, what would you do? If you could change the whole world with your art, what would you do? You are empowered to do this. You can do anything you want to do. You are not alone; you are connected to a network of artists all over the world who are doing the same thing. All it takes is crossing the threshold of the place where you will make it happen and doing it.

A GUIDED IMAGERY EXERCISE TO BECOMING A HEALING ARTIST

This guided imagery is about meeting your healing artist. It is similar to imagery used to meet an inner guide or spirit animal. It is based on listening to the voice of an inner figure, seeing an inner figure who emerges as a helper in your life. The artist within comes from deep within your imagination and is tied to images of the earth and of interconnectedness. When your artist is connected to nature—to an ancient tree, for example—the imagery you make as art is deeply healing to yourself, others, and the earth.

> Close your eyes. Take a couple of deep breaths; let your abdomen rise and fall. Get into your imagery space as you have many times before. Now put yourself on a path. Feel your feet touch the earth. Smell the fresh air; feel the warm breeze on your face. Walk down the path. It goes downhill slightly. The ground is hard and has small stones in the soil. It is solid and secure. Feel the ground and the grass that is on each side of the path. Walk down the path. It crosses a wooden bridge across a rushing stream. The bridge has stout railings. You can hear your feet echo on the bridge like a drumbeat as you walk across. If you need to drop something in the water that you want to get rid of, you can do that now.

> The path now goes upward slightly and comes over a rise. Below you is a large meadow. In the center of the meadow is a grassy circle. Sit in the circle and wait. Now ask for your inner artist to come to you. It is like a spirit figure, coming out of the air or the light. Let the figure appear and walk up to you. It can come from a distance or appear from nowhere. The figure that appears to

you is your artist spirit. It is your inner artist. Let the figure come toward you. Let your artist begin to speak and move. The figure is filled with light. It is free and expansive. It can fly, dance, move, twirl. The artist is there, illuminated in pure light, and you recognize yourself. The artist invites you to stay in the meadow and feel connected to the earth. Your artist reaches out and touches the earth. It has tendrils that reach deep into the earth, the sky, and you and connect it all together.

Feel at one with the trees, the wind, the earth, the stars. Feel your body as the earth. Feel your own body as her body. Feel your bones as her rocks, your flesh as her soil, your muscles as her hillsides, your blood as her rivers. Now feel your blood pulse as she pulses. Feel your breath flow as she breathes, your heart beat as she beats. You are one with the elements. You pulsate inside your own life. You are the earth's body, and in the body there is an awareness of time, of history, of the stories of life in this body. You are connected to the stories of the earth, to the stories of your families, your ancestors. You are part of a living flow. There is a wisdom, a capacity to age and die, to be born and live at once. There is an innate wisdom capacity that comes out from the earth. The power to be formed, to heal, to give birth, to regenerate cells. You are the constant regeneration of healing cells flowing from the earth. You become aware of this.

If you feel comfortable with it now, let your artist move into your body. The artist is yours, living within you. Let the artist in if it feels right. Let the artist move into your body. There is a moment of elation, levity, empowerment. Now you have the power to generate energy in forms, in creative ways. To take it deeper, let the artist merge with the innate healer within your body; let it blend with your body's healing capacity. Then the artist becomes the voice for your body to speak, to teach itself. The artist takes your body to become the poet, the dancer, the painter. As your body moves into the dance, as you take yourself into the flow, the spirit and the body merge and a transformation occurs. You know who you are. You know what you need to do. You wake up and see out of your own eyes. You are a witness to your own life. You create your own life as a healing piece of work.

Now stand up and leave the meadow. The path goes out of the far side, and you can walk further down the path. It leads to the edge of an ancient forest of old-growth trees. Stand at the edge of the forest by a great ancient tree. Find a tree that speaks to you and tells you to come to it. Now put your hand on the tree. Touch its rough bark. Feel its warmth, its life. Now imagine that when you put your hand on the tree, you spiral deep into the spiral of your own being. You spiral deep inside yourself, into your heart. And inside your body, your heart opens with wings. A spirit eye opens within you and sees this experience. It witnesses you becoming the healing artist. Now lift up your hand. Take it off the tree. As you lift up your hand, see that out of your hand come gifts. There are gifts of poems, of paintings, of dances. And you raise your hand and the gifts fly out like birds. You give the gifts away. These are your gifts of love that make you a healing artist. When you touch the tree, become the tree, you are within the body of the tree. You have roots in the earth, you reach for the sun, you take water from the earth, nourishment from the earth, and you nourish the earth with your gifts.

In the tree, there are concentric circles, spirals, the essence of the beingness. It is being with life itself. When you go into this space you are deep. You are deep into the space where you fly. You grow wings; you are like a Buddha opening his eyes for the first time. You see. You become aware of yourself. You see that as the tree grows, it is perfect. As it reaches up into the sun and blossoms with flowers and leaves, they are the creative manifes-

tation of the tree. Each leaf is a gift that drops to the earth like your art. These are gifts we share; they blow away from us like leaves in the wind. We let go of our art; it is a detachment.

Now walk back the way you came. Your body is now different; it is lighter, more powerful. Walk back to the meadow, then to the bridge, then to where you are now. Bring your inner artist with you. Let it still be in touch with your inner healer. Bring the connectedness with you. Bring the spirit of the tree with you. Now move your feet. Look around you. You are now a healing artist. You can make art and give it away. You can make art to heal the earth.

ELEVEN

How Professional Artists Use Art to Heal Themselves, Others, and the Earth

For many years, the field of art and healing has been made up of two different worlds. First, there was the world of the artists working with patients in hospital programs. Second, there was the world of the professional artist making healing art in the studio and in the community. For a long time these worlds were separate. Professional artists did not bring their art to the hospital, and if they worked with patients it was outside the realm of medicine. Physicians did not see the professional artist as a healer. The separation is no longer real or complete. Art and healing are one, and the artist healer is one figure again. The professional artist is now a recognized healer.

The artists we talk about in this chapter have devoted their lives to healing art. These artists are contemporary shamans in that they have taken on the role of being specialists in seeing the soul and portraying it in art to heal. These artists have gone far into a world of inner visions, and they see more deeply. They have perfected techniques that have made their work more powerful and intricate. Their healing art can be thought of as "advanced therapeutic practices" that are inspiring for each of us.

The works these artists create can be intimidating to people who are just beginning to make healing art. It is professional art, and its technical skill often comes from years of training and a lifetime of application. Please don't be intimidated by their art. Instead, realize that their work can be a guide to people starting to heal themselves with art. As you will see from their stories, each artist is also an ordinary person whose story is the same as our story, whose lessons are applicable to all of us.

The first group of artists we will look at are those who have had an illness or a life crisis and started making art in their own studio to heal themselves. Then they became professional artists and devoted their lives to making healing art. Another group in this section are men and women who had been serious and often well-known artists before they became ill and who used their illness to change the focus of their art to healing.

Hollis Sigler Talks about Painting and Breast Cancer

Hollis Sigler is a breast cancer survivor who was a respected painter before she became ill. She was a leader in the feminist art movement, painting scenes about her own life as a woman. After her diagnosis she created a series of paintings that chronicled her inner life with breast cancer. Her work expressed her thoughts about her illness and her anger at the way society views women with breast cancer. Her paintings evoked a sense of vulnerability, of isolation, and sometimes, of waning hope.

The exhibition of her works has toured hundreds of hospitals nationwide and has even been shown at the United States Congress. It has been moving and transformative to women with and without cancer. Women with breast cancer realize that they are not alone in having frightening images of their illness. These stories inform both the clinicians who are committed to facilitating healing and the healing artists. Hollis Sigler has lived with breast cancer for many years. We deeply honor her pioneering work, which communicates so much to all of us. She may be the best-known healing artist today.

Hollis says:

I started out doing the breast cancer artwork as therapy for myself. I was keeping diaries of my experience, and it gave me a handle on what I was feeling about things. It showed me a reflection of my feelings and helped me cope with life. For me, that was its healing experience: the therapeutic quality of letting me have a dialogue with myself about my experience. I think all art is therapy in the end. People will disagree with me, but I think anybody who makes art is in the process of dialoging about their thoughts and their feelings, and therefore the art manifests in a language that they can reflect on.

I felt better, more whole, more complete, through the experience of making art. It helped me understand some of my most painful feelings. I believe that being in touch with yourself and your feelings is a healthy thing to do, so being a visual artist is very beneficial in terms of healing. It helps me cope, and I believe it does have a major effect on healing my breast cancer.

Viewing the work helps give people a voice to their own experience, which is very healing to them. They say, "Oh yes, this is my experience." My art has the ability to include people. In my paintings, I don't talk much as an "I." I talk as a "we." So it is hopefully including others in the dialogue. It helps other women with breast cancer find their voice and be included. My intent is to inform, to talk about my experience and share it with others who have had the experience. It is also to let people know they are not alone. We are a community of women in the process of healing ourselves. It is a process that they can be involved in by making art. They can find their own voice.

When I make art, I have a sensation of great satisfaction; it is very meditative. It is a complete sense of self. In the process of making art, I get transported, moved into another realm that I find very, very relaxing. For me, art making is transporting. I can get out the feelings and have them out there to see. I can encapsulate them and examine them. That was part of the motivation when the initial pieces were made. I was waiting for tests, in limbo, with no past and no future. The present was all-encompassing. Putting it on paper helped me deal with it. It always helped me in crises to put it out there.

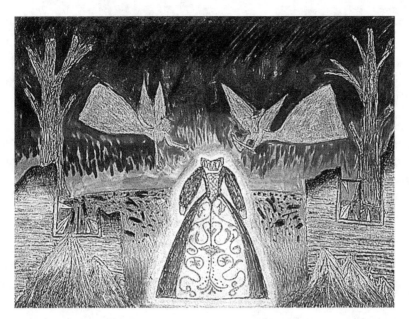

Hollis Sigler, *Hope Again Reigns in the Hearts of Women*. Hollis is a painter who has lived with breast cancer. She is one of the best-known painters in art and healing. She says, "In losing a breast, there is a sense of loss. It is a feeling I own only to myself. But fear of recurrence took hold of my life. The illusion of fear was lost when I encountered my cancer for the third time. There is nothing to lose now."

VISIONARY ARTISTS

Visionary artists make art that is deeply healing to themselves and to the viewer. Studio artists who are visionary artists are absorbed in a creative process so completely that they are merged with visionary space. Visionary artists see deeply into the spirit world. They journey between worlds and bring images out from the spirit world and work them into their paintings.

Alex Grey, a New York painter, is one of the leading visionary artists alive today. He goes deep into a meditative state and brings out images of exceptional beauty and light to share with us. He has created a large installation piece called *Sacred Mirrors* that reveals the beauty of body and soul and allows us to see how we are all connected to nature and to one another. His figures show deep spiritual realms of consciousness, the unity of male and female, the wings of spirit flying, and the peaceful and wrathful aspects of human existence. He portrays worlds that he can see more deeply than most of us, worlds that most of us cannot see at all but know are there.

His pieces are deeply healing and are often used by cancer patients as meditations. Many patients say that his portrayals of space, energy, and healing correspond to their own visions during healing meditations. The pieces were assembled in a book, *Sacred Mirrors*, which is used for healing by people with illnesses as well as by seekers on a spiritual path. He is part of the movement that is bringing art back to its roots as a transformative force. He is a true visionary artist in the tradition of sacred artists throughout history.

An Alex Grey painting draws you in and engages you in a way that can be more intense than some "real" scenes. It accesses your imagination more than a real place might, especially if the place is one you have seen over and over again and are habituated to. The painting magnifies the image and brings it to our fullest attention. Visionary artists convey a spiritual vision, sharing with us their enhanced vision.

Alex Grey believes that visionary artists are people who see the deepest brightness they can see after a lifetime of practice. And then, with the intent to heal, they bring the spiritual vision out to share with the community. That is what all healing artists do. The artists birth the spirit into form with their hands, eyes, and dedication. They give you the gift of their undying passion and commitment to what they do. Visionary artists make spiritual and religious art for a community, and it is their vision that lasts through the ages or changing times. They make images that will speak to the soul and are truly universal.

Alex Grey Talks about Visionary Art

The interconnectedness of body, mind, and spirit became the premier subject for my artwork. That was brought home when I had the psychedelic experience of the universal mind lattice. That was not an art event specifically, but it was a transpersonal experience, the revelation of a strata of being, that I had not previously experienced or known about. It showed me a realm of complete interconnectedness with all beings and things via a love energy that was in an infinite, omnidirectional grid, a sort of fountain-drain, a toroidal shape. Each being and thing was one of the cells interlocked in this ongoing network. It was there with totally no reference point to the external world or external reality—it was all the energetic realm and it felt like the total bedrock of reality. It was this scaffolding of creation that the dreamlike world of mundane manifestation was draped over. It felt like a veil had been stripped away and I was seeing the way things really were. It was beyond time; it was beyond, and it changed my entire point of view about what we are.

I came back from that experience and looked at my wife, Allison. She was looking at me, and I said, "It was the most amazing space—we're there, we're always there. It's just—I've never seen it before. It's where we'll go when we die; it's what I was before I was born." She said, "Yes, I know . . . and it looked like this," and she started drawing it and it was the same space. She saw the same transpersonal space at the same time I did and that just drove it home to me. I'm not saying that that's it, and that's the only space. But it was my initiation into the mystic headspace that I feel is profoundly true. And it did change my outlook on life and spirit.

I felt profoundly grateful for the experience. Afterwards, Allison and I felt that there's nothing else more important to make artwork about. We felt that we had to make art about our interconnectedness and this realm of loving energy we all share. This was something for us to base our lives on. So from that experience, *Sacred Mirrors* started to gel.

Alex Grey's Advice on Making Visionary Art

I think that there are definitely ways you can reach into the psyche, to the most potent visions that you have, and externalize them. I think that in a way, it's more important that the work be heartfelt than that it be greatly skillful. Skillful means can be developed, and I'm not denigrating technical proficiency. I think it's very important, but I think that finding your own personal and universal truth of where you are right now is what is worth making art about. To give yourself the permission to have confidence enough to pick up that pencil or crayon or paintbrush and make the mark out of your own heart and soul, that can be nothing but healing in itself. Keep praying, you know; pray to whatever spiritual source you feel aligned with and look inside and make the work directly from that. That's as simple as I can say it.

ARTISTS MAKING ART TO HEAL OTHER PEOPLE

The second group we'll discuss are professional artists who make art to heal others who are ill or in the middle of life crises. These artists can work with groups of people in workshops or classes or work one-on-one. They make art to heal the community, to heal a neighborhood, to heal certain groups of people, to heal race relations, to create peace, to heal prejudice. In neighborhood art projects, they often involve groups of people in creativity that increases self-esteem, a sense of empowerment, and a drive to change, while at the same time achieving neighborhood beautification. The projects can be done in schools, hospitals, community centers, or parks.

Christiane Corbat is an artist who lives in Providence, Rhode Island. She was a sculptor who made static figures. After a period of great darkness and suffering in her life, she made a casting of her own body. She found the process and the sculpture to be deeply healing and transformational. She then began to make body-casting sculpture with people who had physical or emotional illnesses or were seeking spiritual growth. She made a series of sculptures called *Amazons* for women with breast cancer. From Christiane's sculptures, women could see themselves as beautiful. Often they would take the sculpture home and use it as part of a healing meditation. In one sculpture, the sutures around the mastectomy were to be plucked as harp strings to turn the suffering into music. In past years, Christiane has made body castings of people with heart disease, organ transplants, asthma, and other diseases. Each piece of art gives the person a new transformative view of themselves or their illness. Her sculpture is a new type of studio art: art made with intent to heal another person.

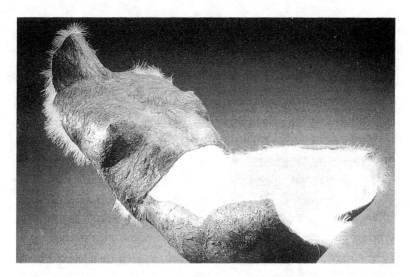

Christiane Corbat, *Open Woman*. Christiane is a master at making art to heal others. She is a healing artist extraordinaire. She says, "The *Open Woman* was my first figure piece. I made it as a self-portrait; a woman as a passage or conduit in which inner and outer space are equally important. This is a piece about emotional and psychological openness, but I use the body to evoke the vulnerability of such an act. I made her totally unguarded, because she needs no defense. My thought was that the entire universe could pass through her and leave her unharmed; nourish her, excite her, and fill her with awe. She is reclined, receptive. I filled her with white feathers to indicate her tender insides and to capture the outside light. I covered her with paper from a wasp nest, a material also taken from nature, to announce her wildness and her natural beauty. The very act of making this piece transformed me. All subsequent pieces have been made with the intent to transform myself or others because of the empowerment I experience by becoming the open woman."

Christiane's process is simple, elegant, and completely extraordinary at once. People are often referred to her by physicians. She talks to the person who comes to her, and together they see a vision. The vision comes out of the simple sharing of stories of the lived experience of the person's illness. Together they see the spirit of how the person will transform. Then Christiane makes a casting of the person's body. The piece of art embodies the transformation, is the transformed form, and the person's participation helps make the process happen. Christiane herself is transformed, too. She is now the embodied shaman, the one who sees the transformation, manifests it, and makes it happen. She is an artist healer, a contemporary shaman, an exceptional woman.

Christiane Corbat Tells Us about How She Makes Art to Heal Others

My intent when I work with people is to help them to access their healing so that they become aware of it. I can make the image that will help them to get on that wavelength or move in that direction. We cast their bodies to see the change that will happen and help it happen. In *A Fine Line between Hope and Despair,* made with a man named Larry who was dealing with heart disease, it was the balancing act with the scale. It was our consciously pushing down on hope, which was light as a feather, and pushing up despair, which was those two very heavy pieces of metal, that let him control it himself. He becomes the one who can balance his life.

We gave him an image that he could use to make hope carry the day. He could use it on a regular basis when he needed it. The casting process was very similar to having an angiogram in that it took place in stillness. Our process will help him prepare for the medical process that he's going to have done on a regular basis. Maybe peace and control will come to him as he is lying there on that table now that he's doing the balancing act. I think it's very important to give people a myth that they can carry when they are going through a crisis or a crucial moment. If you can be a hero or heroine or you can have a power animal, that ideal helps give you a tremendous amount of power.

I have always found that what's very important is to involve all the loved ones of the person I'm doing the piece with. And so with Larry, I invited him to bring whomever he wanted, and he brought his whole family. He brought his wife, his daughter, her husband, his son and his fiancee, and a brother-in-law. And everybody partook of this event, and then I had them actually cast their arms to put inside his body cavity, into the chest, where his heart needed help and so they physically became part of this. He was able to meta-phorically, through this piece, explain exactly how he felt about them, which had been very difficult and it just opened up huge areas for everybody—communication, closeness, intimacy.

How Healing Art Changes Your Life

Christiane Corbat says, in making healing art, you become yourself. You are who you are, but more so. You are fully there and able to do anything you want to without fear, even face your own death. You are changed totally. You are a different person. You become the shaman, the one who can make change, the one who can turn spirit into matter. For you now, all of life is open, it is an adventure. You meet people, see them as wonderful, as beautiful. You are fully present in the moment. You are just who you are being alive. You know why you are here and what you are meant to do and you do it with total love. The healing art flows from you with love and you are only Her song on earth.

Christiane describes to us how art has changed her life.

> Now, since I've been making art this way, I have to tell you that my life has changed radically. I'm living just the most extraordinary life that I could ever have imagined, and perhaps that's one of the things about healing art. It heals all the places in you that need healing; it fills those places up and it makes it possible for you to give this to the rest of the community. I became fully myself. I was in a place of great crisis and great pain and I didn't know how to get unstuck, and I turned to my art. I turned to it, saying, "You've always been my way of expression—what can I do?" And it healed me. It healed me and I am the same but I am more so in every way and I can do things I could never have done before. I am just more fully, fully me and can be myself in all directions. That's a wonderful way to live.

STARTING A HEALING ART GROUP

Many artists work with individuals in the community in informal situations, say in their studios or homes. Annie Pais is a painter in Florida who set up a studio in her home and created a community of women who came together to make art. As she worked with them, she realized that the making of art was a meditation, that it was a way for the women who came to paint to get deeper into their own lives. She saw that they made art to deal with the issues of their lives and to empower themselves, and that by working together in a creative process, there was more energy. In Annie's own process, she believed that art was spirit becoming matter. She herself had used art as prayer, as meditation. She believed that by using the art as a creative process for healing, it would be profoundly powerful. What evolved was that the group started doing ceremony and ritual together. One woman who was pregnant would make art of pregnant women; another woman dealing with her beauty did art of flowers. As a collective, all the pieces of art began to weave a story together.

This healing art group had started as a simple art class where she had invited women to get together and make art in her home. It turned into a woman's healing group that used art to heal. Next, Annie began to work with women who are surviving cancer. She became increasingly involved with people who see themselves as healing. She now does art workshops with cancer survivors. They rent a beach house together and just make art for a week. They have a healing artist's retreat, which evolved out of an informal process. It emerged out of a need, as she saw that the art was healing. She continued because she was committed in her own path.

With Annie, much of the healing process centered around painting what the artists loved. She encouraged people to paint what they were in love with. She taught them to look at art as a way of falling deeper in love with the things in life around them. She would paint beautiful still lifes of things she loved and get people to look around their own lives for things that they loved. She painted the magnolias, the blue heron, her living room furniture. It was very ordinary and beautiful. Work like Annie's shows us that there are numerous ways to do art and healing with others. It does not have to be in a hospital program or even with patients; it can be in any way you see yourself in the community working as a healing artist. Her work also shows us that you do not need to know what you are doing in advance. It will grow by itself.

MEDICINE ART

Medicine art is art that radiates power to heal. When the Yoruba of Africa create fertility dolls, they make them and pray for fertility in one process. It is believed that the prayers go up to the spirit, and the spirit actually comes down into the doll. When the Yoruba make twin dolls to keep babies together, they are treated as if they are alive, and the twins are fed and cared for. When the objects are treated as alive, they become alive to the person and are seen as filled with energy. They become infused with life and spirit. People believed that spirit resides in them. Healing artists make objects that become alive with spirit. A Maori woodcarver told us that his carvings radiate power. Maori tradition says that the figures have energy fields that affect the world around them. The carver believes that his figures heal by changing the air and molecules. He said that they would work even if the people did not know the legends the piece represented. The Tibetan Buddhists believe that art is an incarnation of the deity on earth, that art is sacred as a presence and powerful in itself. They believe that the deity comes into the piece and gives it power.

Sandy Carlson is a Florida sculptor who makes spirit dolls. She is a contemporary shamanic image maker. She believes that she makes form that the spirit comes into so that the form embodies the spirit. Her art gives the spirit a place to rest and a home. Her pieces of art become your friends; they become speakers and seers in your life. The objects themselves carve out destiny; they bring certain energies into your life. They are alive and rich. A woman who lives with one of her figures says,

> When I first bought the Kali spirit doll, the goddess came home with me. My life became involved with death and rebirth. It was like the spirit was in the house and brought that powerful energy into my life. She kept me company in my sadness and when it was over she took my sadness. She keeps the treasure of the memory of my sadness. I don't have to keep it in my body anymore. I can release it. If you let go of the anger, you don't have to feel the pain and sadness anymore. The doll can hold the sadness in space and time. It no longer hurts you. When I was the most sad, I could see I was sad, and I am changed now.

The art can be abstract or a portrait. The subject is not important. It is what it brings out in you that heals. The forms belong with you; they live a life with you. They are transformative in themselves and have their own power.

Medicine art objects have been made with the purpose of healing. Any art that comes into your life can change your life; it is imagery that is powerful. Images that are of a visionary landscape make the visionary world real. They bring the visionary world into your life. An image of a deity or of Christ or Buddha brings the holy spirit of that being into your life. Beauty illuminates your life when you hang a painting filled with radiant beauty. Calm comes into your life when you hang a painting that is calming. Painful images brought into your life stir up difficult emotions. You are attracted to what you recognize.

ARTISTS WHO USE ART TO HEAL THE EARTH

The third group of artists are those who use art to heal the earth. They believe that the earth is alive and is presently disrupted and needs to be healed. They believe that making art in watersheds, or mountains, or dry lake beds changes the energy and heals. Making earth art is deeply transformative to the artists. They feel a sense of connection to the earth that is beautiful and sacred. In fact, many of these artists believe that the earth speaks to them through art. These artists receive images from the earth to make art that heals the earth. It is as if she is speaking to them for herself. All healing artists believe that the earth is helping them heal, but the artists who heal the earth live within the earth's voice and hear her song.

To be any type of healing artist, it is important to ground yourself in the living earth, to ground yourself in the sacred places where you live. It is important to see the sacred places on the earth around you as places that nourish you and give you energy. Each place that you live in has a place that is sacred and full of power. In Gainesville, Florida, where AIM is located, it is the springs; in Marin County, California, the home of Anna Halprin's Tamalpa Institute and Michael's Art As A Healing Force, it is Mount Tamalpais. In Providence, Rhode Island, where Christiane Corbat makes her healing body castings, it is the ocean. Find the sacred places around you and go deeply into them and feel the energy from within. Go to the sacred springs, the rocks, the mountains, the ocean, the caves, the old trees.

It is important for all healing artists to be deeply connected to the earth. Nature is in a constant creative process. Nature is always giving birth and taking its life back into its body. Nature tells you that what you are doing as a healing artist is totally natural. Making art is what nature does; making art to heal is what nature is. You go to the sacred places near where you live to meditate and nourish and heal. They inform you of what is real in the change of seasons, in the changing light, and in the shadows and the darkness. They create the opportunity for you to know where you are. The path you are on is the path you are on, and the sacred places in nature remind you that you are deeply alive and creative as you are.

The life of a healing artist is the same as a vision quest. A vision quest was a ceremony done by some Native American peoples in which young people went into nature to find themselves. They sat for days in a secluded place and waited for a spirit animal or voice to come to them and tell them who they were or what they were to do on earth. The vision quest was about finding their own spirit and helping others. It was about listening to the voices of the earth and the ancient ones. Becoming a healing artist or healing yourself with art is also about making your life a sacred vision quest. It is also about finding out who you are and what you are to do here.

As a healing artist, your life is a vision quest—literally, a quest for visions. Your own personal life is informing you in every way. You have shifted from an ordinary person who is only occupied with the dailiness of material things to someone who is concentrating on healing yourself, healing another, or healing the earth. The work is connected to your own life. It comes out of your life, and as you see your art emerge, you know that everything is perfect as it is, that it will bring you to where you are. The work is difficult because often you will fall back on yourself for support, and sometimes you'll have to keep reminding yourself how profound and sacred the work is. Alex Grey says that if you don't doubt this work occasionally, you are not going deep enough into it. Doubt is facing the opposites, the tension, of life. When you go deeply into your visions you feel the dark even as you are in the light.

So to ground yourself in this work, look to the earth. You can do sacred pilgrimages, be alone, meditate with the earth, do an intentional healing of the earth. We believe that all healing art is healing the earth. Whenever you heal yourself or heal another, you heal the earth as well. You can canoe down a river or stand on a temple mound and realize you have been touched by the earth. Your spirit soars, and you pray with the intention of being with the earth.

Anouk's Path of the Feather

One day, Anouk arrived. She told us she was on the "path of the feather." She was a sculptor and jeweler from Montreal, Canada, and she came to the AIM program at Shands Hospital to make healing art. She had been to the rivers and had collected rocks. She brought these "rock people" to the bedsides of children with cancer. She told the children stories about Native American medicine, and she had the children paint the rocks the five different colors of the medicine wheel. Each color evoked one element of the medicine wheel—yellow for change, red for healing, blue for passion, black for grounding, green for soaring.

Then she collected the rocks from all the children and arranged them in a circle in the center of the hospital sun terrace. She built a sacred medicine wheel painted by the children with cancer. She had everyone who came by pray to heal each person who had painted the rocks and do imagery to bring up a collective energy to spiral from the earth up to the sky. She believed that the raising of the energy healed the earth. She merged healing the children with healing the earth. The rocks stayed in place for three weeks in this busy terrace in the middle of the medical center. It was healing art to heal the patients, the staff, and the medical center itself. It created a space in the heart of the hospital that was healing art.

It was her idea to make art at the bedside and then do the ritual in the sun terrace. It was an act of boldness and fearlessness in her life as a person and as an artist. The first day she came to the hospital, she walked into a patient's room and asked the person to draw with her. She did not know the patient was blind, and she felt terrible when she realized it. She was embarrassed, shy, and upset, and she had to get all her energy up to keep working in the hospital. Within six weeks she was so brave that she could create her story of the healing medicine wheel of rocks. Anouk as an artist emerged from afar, came in, put her healing artistry to work, and then was gone. It was as simple as that. We must create openings for people like this.

Vijali Talks about Healing the Earth

Vijali is an earth artist who heals with the light that comes from within her heart. She had been a studio painter in Los Angeles and had a vision that she should go to the mountains and become a hermit. She moved up to a tiny trailer in the mountains outside of Los Angeles and lived alone. There the rocks spoke to her. A rock opened and showed her how to look within. She saw there that she was to go around the earth and stay with people and make art to heal. She went to nine countries in seven years in her World Wheel project. In each country she would ask three questions: What is your essence? What is holding you back from being it (that is, what is your illness)? And what can you do to achieve who you are (that is, what is your healing)? Then, with the local people, she would do an earth carving or performance piece that embodied the answers to the questions. She would live with the people for months and fall in love with them and their lives. She would heal them as a community by making the piece with them and sharing in their healing.

Vijali says:

> My intention in my work now is to heal the planet. Of course, we are the planet—we are part of the planet. All this dissension, wars, bloodshed around the world, we are it too. There is intention in my preparation for the next World Wheel. I want to call for a global cease-fire for forty-eight hours. There is an intention of getting peace into the world, peace into each individual's life, which I think is the only way to have world peace. We are on the way to a world transformation, so I am working on a very personal level as well as on a global level with the intention of healing. My work right now is global healing.
>
> Who am I? I'm just light and space, with red mud splattered on it. When I speak of art, I don't just mean paintbrushes. I mean the whole of life—where you go, how you sit, how you do everything. Everything is part of that gesture of creating. Every thought we have has an effect on the whole galaxy, the whole cosmos. So everything is important, everything is sacred, and everything is

ritual. And ritual has an effect on people, so every part of every gesture is having an effect.

There is no separation for me between art and prayer. No, the art is truly the prayer; there is absolutely no separation. The prayer, when you make a prayer, is words. The words are vibration or sound, even if you're thinking and nothing is said out loud. That thought itself is creating a particular vibration, and on some level, even that thought is a sound. The same thing is true with sculpture. As you're carving the sculpture, it's saying something; it is a vibration that is sent out into the world. It is prayer.

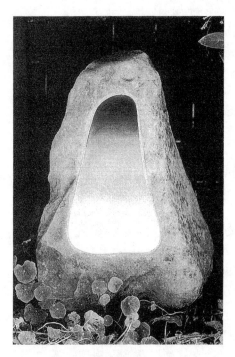

Vijali, *Spirit within Matter*. Vijali is an earth artist who does ceremonies and rituals to heal the earth. "The stone was like a doorway, and I just saw this burst of light. It seemed to connect everything. The stone represented my body, my flesh, the earth itself. That was the moment when I started working. I felt my own body, my spirit, my mind coming into a harmony. After that happened I was healing. I saw there was no separation."

In the next World Wheel, I'm going to have just one question. The next World Wheel will be dedicated to the children of the world because I feel this next period will be for them; they will be inheriting this world. I feel they are very important and so I'm going to ask them particularly, "How can you bring peace into the world?" I'm going to videotape the children around the world and have them answer that question. I'm going to carry a book because some children will be too young to verbalize their answer, and I will have them draw it in my book. I will have people write in their own script and the children draw their answers.

You know, we're being healed in the process of everyone else being healed. I was such a damaged child; and I think that if the child that I was could be happy, filled with joy, the way I am now, anyone can be healed. I couldn't read until I was thirteen years old, and people would talk to me and I was so shy that I couldn't look up. I thought, "They must be talking to someone else, someone in back of me," so I wouldn't even say a word, and people would be talking to me. At school, they thought I was deaf because I couldn't answer. They kept having my ears examined because I wouldn't respond. I was such a mess and in so much pain internally.

One reason I am doing the World Wheel is that I didn't have a family, so I keep looking for other ways to have a family. Now I have a global family. The art really helped me, because I was always drawing, even from the age of two, even if I couldn't communicate very well with people. The art led me into the world and into my own healing and the healing of others.

Vijali's Advice on How to Heal with Art

Well, I would say to really follow your heart and do what you really love. And never make decisions, which parents are always telling kids to do, about the practical (you know, "Do this job because you're going to make money and it's more practical). But do what you really want to. Go and paint, or if you want to work with children do that, because that's the clue from the inside to what is really right. It is the clue to how you yourself will unfold, and what would be really healing for you. And what heals you is the healing you do for other people in the world. It's your contribution to the world. So follow your own inner voice, really connect with your own guru, not a guru or a teacher from outside. You can learn tools from teachers, but . . .

You can meditate. Take time to be alone, to make contact. By just hanging out with yourself in nature, you can become attuned to yourself and your world. We all have this ability; we just don't pay attention to it. You know, it's like our culture tells us not to daydream. You might be sitting in school and looking out the window and daydreaming, but that's supposed to be bad because you're supposed to be writing down what the teacher is saying. But we have to hear these little feelings that float up. We just have to follow those little moments that really tell us what is right for us to do. Then, step-by-step, we are led into our own healing and way of being.

DOING RITUAL ON SACRED SITES TO HEAL

Artists and healers are finding that sacred sites are important healing resources for healing themselves, others, and the earth. Healers are taking patients to sacred sites to heal them, and artists are going to sacred sites to make healing art and do intentional healing rituals. There are sacred sites in your backyard and in ancient stone circles; they are both gifts to the healing artist.

Sacred sites play a major role in art and healing. The energies they hold from the earth and the rituals done in the past flow up into us to empower us deeply. Sacred sites are most often situated near rivers, caves, springs, mountains, ancient trees, or the sea. And the energy of these earth forces comes up into our body, mind, and spirit to make any healing more effective. The ancient ones who did the rituals to heal in the distant past come to us in visions and speak to us and give us their power, too. The thought forms of the ancient healers are around these sites, and we can feel them and they come into us. People have found places of power that follow a line across an area; this is called a ley line. Often there are churches, ancient stone circles, springs, caves, mountains, and ancient trees on these ley lines. In Great Britain, there are ley lines that go from one end of the country to the other. Healers and artists do ritual on these lines to heal.

Artist healers now do rituals in sacred sites all over the world. They do rituals at sacred springs, ancient trees, mountains, stone circles, and temple mounds. They use sacred sites to empower them in their work as artist healers. Each place, every community and wild area, has its sacred sites. Artist healers are now finding and creating their own sacred sites through ritual. Vijali, in her World Wheel, has created a ring of sacred sites around the earth. By making healing art with communities in nine countries around the world she made new sites that people can visit and use for healing ritual. Ritual is embodied in multimedia healing art. It is a performance piece done with sacred intent to heal. It is the oldest art and the oldest healing. It uses dance, music, visual arts, and storytelling all at once to produce transformation. Many healing artists use ritual in sacred sites with any other healing art that they are doing at the time. The ritual enhances the art they are making. Sacred sites are an important resource for artist healers in their work.

MENDING THE HEART NET; PUTTING IT ALL TOGETHER

More and more of us are putting it all together, making healing art to heal ourselves, others, and the earth all at once. Alex Grey did a performance art piece at Shands Hospital, Gainesville, which did this. His piece, *Mending the Heart Net*, was done to heal himself, his family, the patients in the hospital, their families, the hospital staff, the hospital itself, art, medicine, the community, and the earth. *Mending the Heart Net* became the focus of several weeks of ritual for the artists in the community, for a major art and healing conference, and for people coming into Shands Hospital. It truly was about putting it all together.

Mending the Heart Net was a sacred ritual. It was the first performance art piece done in a medical center by a major performance artist. Its occurrence changed the hospital's sterile space into a sacred celebratory space where love and healing could be manifest with intent. Its beauty and symbolism were transformative to everyone in the community who came and participated.

The piece consisted of a heart made of fabric with the earth and continents sewn on it. It had an eye in the center of the heart and a paintbrush surrounded with a serpent on top of the heart. Around the heart were fabric arms and hands with a heart sewn on each palm. The hands even had fingernails. Surrounding the heart was a rope net that extended about twenty feet in each direction. The piece was made by Alex and Allison before they came to Gainesville and was assembled on-site in the hospital atrium in front of patients, family, and staff as they walked by or sat and watched.

The piece was done in the main entryway of Shands Hospital, the main teaching hospital of the University of Florida Medical Center. Most of the patients and staff go through the entryway many times a day. A table set up

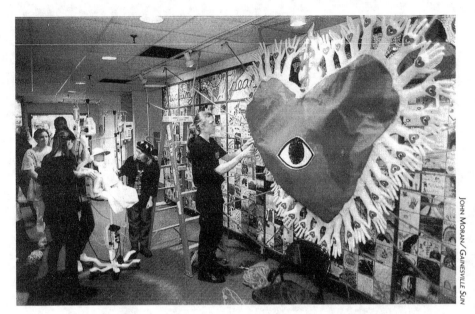

Alex Grey, *Mending the Heart Net*. *Mending the Heart Net* was a performance piece done in the atrium of Shands Hospital on Valentine's Day, 1997. It was the first major piece of performance art done in a hospital to heal. Each person who passed by was invited to write wishes or prayers for healing, and to hang the wishes on the heart net. The process of making the piece as a community brought local artists, healers, patients, and staff together for this special occasion.

in front of the piece had cut-up bandages and pens on it. A sign invited everyone to write a prayer on a bandage for someone who was ill or to write their heart's desire. As patients, staff, visitors, and family members came in, they wrote their prayers or wishes on the cut bandages. The bandages were then pinned to a heart and tied individually to the web. By the end of the day, the web was covered with prayers. The prayers said everything from "please heal my mother of cancer we love her" to "may peace come on earth." They were heartfelt and wonderful. The moment of writing the prayer was surprising and magical for everyone. So many people coming in to face difficult times could stop for a moment and be with others and pray with intent. While people wrote their prayers, live music was played by musicians on a piano, a harp, and guitars.

All afternoon people wrote their prayers and talked to Alex, Allison, their young daughter, Zena, and the AIM artists. Children in wheelchairs were brought down from their rooms by their parents to see the huge heart. At the end of the day, Alex , Allison, and Zena sat in front of the heart, and Alex read a poem. The performance was the making of the heart web and the writing and hanging of the prayers. It gave patients, staff, and families the opportunity to pray with intent and see their prayers in a net with others.

Arts In Medicine artists took the piece down in a ritual after two weeks. Then, two of the artists read the prayers out loud for a whole week as a chant and typed them up so that they could be shown to the hospital administrators. They then were taken to a nearby spring and the artists did a healing ritual. One artist portrayed the old woman of the springs, and she read the prayers and gave the bandages, now tied together in a long rope, to the other artists. Each artist read the prayers they were holding out loud. The artists then went down the river in canoes and stopped in a meadow with a huge ancient tree. The tree had been hit by lightning, and its center was burned out. To the artists, it symbolized the creative fire within each of them, the power of lightning to open their hearts. Each artist entered the tree and prayed for his or her healing artist to emerge, be filled with passion, and be strong. They then buried the prayers in the earth in the center of the tree. Later the artists had a celebration and honored one another as healing artists.

This piece was a ritual to heal that can be done in any medical center by anyone. Of course, Alex, Allison, and Zena are extraordinary, but we all can do this, too. Giving people who visit a hospital the opportunity to write out a prayer is very beautiful and transformative. Giving the artists in the program the opportunity to come together in ritual is also valuable.

Alex Grey's Visualization to Mend the Heart Net

You can participate in Alex and Allison's performance ritual by looking at the photo of the heart net and by doing the imagery exercise. As you do it you can imagine that you are healing yourself, others, and the earth.

> *Close your eyes. Breathe deeply and regularly. Relax and let go*
> *of tensions. When you are ready, bring your attention to your*

own heart center. Many religions point to the heart center as the dwelling place of the soul. Feel the warm glow and loving presence in your own heart center. Now, using your imagination, project a beam of light from your own heart center out to the symbol of the heart net. Sense the commingling of energy with the heart of the world, a network of love that links all beings and things. Hands of light reach out from the heart net to help activate all healing and positive intentions. See the heart net accomplishing the fulfillment of good aims through thousands of beings performing heart-centered actions. Now, having seen your own love energy connected with an infinite network of love energy, it is time to bring the power of the heart net back into your own body. Imagine that the infinite love energy of the heart net condenses to a point at the center of the eye in the giant world heart. From the eye, a powerful beam of light shoots into your own heart center, filling you with clarity and tremendous healing, loving, creative, energy. All of your soul's energy is returned to your body, even from troubling problems, which may have felt draining. You inwardly promise to use this energy to benefit others.

Alex said, "This event honors the special connections between healing, art, and the spirit of love. At their best, what links art and medicine is that they are both heart-centered offerings of service."

ART AS A DOORWAY TO BRINGING IN SPIRITUAL PRACTICE

The more we look at art and healing, the more we believe that it is deeply tied to the concept of art as spiritual transcendence. Transcendence has to do with going into the place in yourself where the spirit resides and then coming out with spirit in your life. In healing art as a path, you go into the center of your being, where your heart is most open, and then come outward. You go into the moment, within your body, and then go deeper. In healing art as a spiritual path, the way to get into the experience of transcendence is to spiral deeper and deeper into the breath, the movement, the flow of creativity. In this chapter we looked at transcendence, light, healing energy, and the spirit. If you are a person healing yourself with art or an artist making art to heal, this chapter should help you see deeper. In this path, your body becomes totally spacious. Our conception of the body is that within it we are infinite. The body is our doorway to the infinite, to the stars in the universe. Inside us is a meditation space as spacious as the infinite sky. Within yourself, as you go deeper and deeper, you get to a place where your body as you know it no longer exists. In this place, it looks the same as the universe; it is the oneness. She holds you there and sends you back deeply changed. This experience is healing art as transcendence.

Transcendence is going into the oneness. The oneness is critical. The oneness with yourself is when you make art. The oneness with the other person is when you make art together. Then, you slip through the membrane, where you share a moment of being, that is, being with the other person where you are deeply connected. It is most like being in love, you are filled with compassion. You love him or her beyond perfectly, you love the other person into the place where he or she is spirit. That is healing. You see the other person for who he or she is in that moment in time and space. When that person is seen, he or she exists. When the other person is not seen, he or she exists in your prayers. Being seen is being honored. Art is about being seen on a deeper level. It is about being seen for who we really are. Being seen as beauty without judgment. This is critical to the process. Healing cannot take place without honoring the spirit and seeing it. The most profound experience with the healer is when he or she walks into the room and sees deeply who you are and honors your spirit. It is the divine within us being heard and seen. It is the most beautiful gift you can give yourself, another person, or the earth.

CONCLUSION

Transforming the Future: Become a Healing Artist

It is like putting on the mask
of the healing artist
and taking it off.

When you take the mask off
the second time
you realize you are changed
and your world is changed.

In listening to the beautiful stories of the lived experience of art and healing, we hear these themes: Art saved my life. I would not be here if it weren't for my art. Art healed my life. Art healed my illness. Art healed me of my childhood. Art will take us to the future and heal the earth.

And we hear artists and healers tell us that art and healing changes your life. Art and healing tells you who you are. Art and healing lets you be yourself more deeply in all directions. Art and healing takes you elsewhere, away from your suffering. Art and healing lets you see the most brilliant illumination you can find and bring it out for everyone to share. Art and healing lets you fall in love. Art and healing lets you see yourself and others as beautiful. Art and healing lets you bring luminosity to yourself and others. Art and healing is about intent. Art and healing is about trust. Art and healing is about loving Her and hearing Her voice and singing it on earth. Art and healing is about community. Art and healing brings spirituality to art and to healing. Art and healing brings spirit into each of our lives. Art is the most beautiful thing I do except loving my family.

In listening to the stories of the artists doing this work, we hear this advice. To do art and healing, it helps to be present in the moment, totally open, and completely flexible. To do art and healing, it helps to be committed and see ourselves as artist healers. To do art and healing, it helps to be in love with life, with beauty, and with the next moment. When we are artist healers, we are the oldest healers and the oldest artists that exist. We join the tradition of art for transformation and healing. We help the mind, body, and spirit resonate as one. We open our hearts to see the people we work with as magnificent and as our equals, as people we love. We see them, hear them, and honor them by helping them make art and see, hear, and honor themselves. We honor this process with our whole life. We see beauty beyond our dreams in our next breath and in theirs. Healing in the broadest sense is finding and embracing life. In the seeing of others, we see ourselves. It is knowing who we are and what we are to do. It is being born into perfect compassion and grace, into connection and oneness. It is about deeply falling in love with Her and singing Her songs on earth.

For most people, the story of healing yourself begins when you are ill and you exhaust the resources outside of yourself to heal. You reach for art when the loneliness and inner turmoil you experience are still there, when you leave the therapist after the fifty-minute visit or leave the oncologist after chemotherapy and know there is more to healing than what happened to you in that office. You reach for art when you feel you need something else, when you feel angry, sad, miserable, unfulfilled, or depressed. And then you may remember that you have always wanted to be an artist and have never done anything about it. Or you just may be drawn to this work. In the illness, you are self-absorbed and struggling for your own personal survival. You realize that the painting or the dance or the poetry or the journal is the way to be with yourself. Making art is the way to be with the pain and live with it, not in an inability to deal with it but in an engaged process where you form it and are in relationship to it. It takes you out of the darkness and into forms. And in the art, everything suddenly has a relationship with the disease and the illness. The art lets you be with it, not talk about it.

Your art is like a cocoon you spin around yourself. Suddenly after you start, you surround yourself in it, you go into your studio, and you are totally absorbed with it; it merges you with the pain and illness, and one day you pop out of it. You emerge out of it and you can see the cocoon, and you are transformed, and the memory of what you were before you entered the cocoon is the artwork. That is what is left. You can see who you once were and you are now different, and you can fly like a butterfly, and you are beautiful, and you can see who you once were and how beautiful you now are. And you can see how in the making of art you were becoming who you are now. And you realize the depth, the extent, of the change that is possible. The caterpillar does not see the butterfly, but the butterfly can look back and see where they were.

OUR DREAM: AN ARTIST FOR EVERY PATIENT, A PATIENT FOR EVERY ARTIST

It is our hope that every patient will include creative healing in his or her healing journey. We also hope that nursing programs, medical schools, and art schools will include art and healing as a part of their program. And we hope that community artists will be able to expand their world in ever more meaningful ways through service.

Our dream is of every patient making art and an artist for every patient. We hope that all hospitals will fund art programs to enhance the quality of care and that artists will innovatively create forms to make their art transformative. Research needs to be done qualitatively and quantitatively to determine how art heals. More research needs to be done to demonstrate that art improves the quality of life, reduces symptoms, and relieves pain. Important research needs to be done to demonstrate that art lengthens the life of people with life-threatening illness and that it cures illness. This is best done by both artists and providers in a multidisciplinary team approach. This view of the future requires a radical change in consciousness that can be achieved through education and consumer pressure. The changing medical system is looking for therapies that are inexpensive and have tremendous benefit. Because the arts are a self-initiated process, art in healing is cost-effective. The power of these processes lies in the individual. The hope for art and healing lies in our hearts. As artists find that they need to make art to heal and healers find they cannot practice healing without art, art and healing will become one.

A GUIDED IMAGERY EXERCISE OF THE FUTURE OF ART AND HEALING

This imagery is yours. It is for you to fill in from your own imagination. By now you will have images of healing that you love, pictures of yourself as an artist healer, images that heal you, others, and the earth. I will only give you the sketchiest of outlines for you to image on. Bless you as your healing artist. Be well.

We invite you to close your eyes and go anywhere. Go to a healing place, a place where you make art, a place where you live as who you are. See what it looks like, smells like, feels like. Look at the natural landscape that surrounds you, the buildings, if any, the sky, the water, the ground, the trees. Look at the art or sculpture around you, listen to the music, join in the dancing. Read words around you or listen to songs around you. See the community of which you are a part. See your family or friends. See yourself as an artist, as a healer, as yourself fully. See yourself loved perfectly from before the beginning of time to after the end of time. See this become your life. Now open your eyes, and bring this healing vision out with you into your life. What part of it can you live now? What part of it, even the smallest part, can you make come true now?

THE MEDICINE WHEEL WEB

The World Wide Web on the Internet is a way we can all focus our psychic energy in one place at once. If we all picture an image of healing the earth in the traditions of shamanic artist healers, it will happen. We have set up the Medicine Wheel Web on the World Wide Web to help heal ourselves, heal others, and heal the earth with healing art. It is part of our larger Web site at www.artashealing.org. Our Web site has information about the field of art and healing, about conferences, events, and exhibitions, and it lists links to other sites. We hope that each healing artist who reads our site and our book will be part of a collective consciousness of people making art to heal. And we hope that each person who is healing with art will become a part of the Web, too, to share in the healing prayers and help heal.

The Medicine Wheel Web is about becoming an intentional healing part of the consciousness that surrounds the earth. We all join, share our visions, pray as one, and find the other who dreams as we do. Through the noosphere, the consciousness that surrounds the earth, we become one consciousness, with each of our parts still remaining individual. The term *noosphere* was first used by Pierre Teilhard de Chardin, a Jesuit paleontologist, to refer to his concept of a thinking envelope that surrounds the earth and acts as a collective consciousness. Many people realize that the World Wide Web is a noosphere, since through it we can merge and think as one being. We believe that one function of the noosphere is to see the earth and heal her and to receive the thoughts from the universe as it grows and looks back on itself. Our Web site is about becoming intentionally part of the healing noosphere as it self-balances the earth.

Healing artists can make up a living medicine wheel that surrounds the earth. They can be the part of the noosphere that balances and heals. You are healing by just making art. You are a node on the noosphere that is like a cell in the immune system or a cell that can produce growth and regeneration. You are a node in the noosphere that can see into the mind of the universe and be one with it as it grows. The artist creates images, sounds, movements, and poems that resonate in the noosphere all at once. You are like flowers in a spherical wreath around the earth. As you resonate as one, all of us are healed.

We hope that each artist on this wheel will find others who are having the same dreams, bringing in the same images. We hope that anyone who needs to be healed will find others who are doing the work they are involved in. Healing artists who make bears will see other people who have the same dreams and make bear art. You will find your spirit brothers, sisters, and lovers. This is about knowing that you are not alone. You will see that someone believes in you, that you are being seen. This is about seeing you. You are being illuminated in the world so you can see yourself and others can see you, too. That is how the earth is healing herself. As we see ourselves in these moments, the earth is healed. This is about you seeing yourself as a healing artist. This is about being a healing artist with others as a ritual healing act. When an artist becomes part of the living medicine wheel, he or she intentionally becomes part of the noosphere that will heal the earth.

A COLLECTIVE GUIDED IMAGERY EXERCISE TO HEAL YOURSELF, OTHERS, AND THE EARTH

This guided imagery is on our Web site and allows us all to actually image at once.

> Imagine that you are in the center of an immense field of healing energy. As one of the minds around the earth, you are like a star in an immense constellation that is the living being evolving toward God. We believe that if everyone pictured a healing form at once, the earth would heal.

> Blessings to you. Welcome to the spirits of healing, the four directions, the animal spirits, the ancient ones. Call them in to you as you breathe and as you look to each side of you in a prayer. Now make yourself comfortable, take some deep breaths and let your abdomen rise and fall, go to your place of imagery or meditation, go to your place of peace and power.

> Now imagine a web of light that surrounds the earth. It looks like lines of light or pure energy crossing and meeting at nodes that light up and explode with love. Now imagine that you are one intersection, one node of exploding light and love, for each of us as a healing artist is only alive as the node lights up and holds

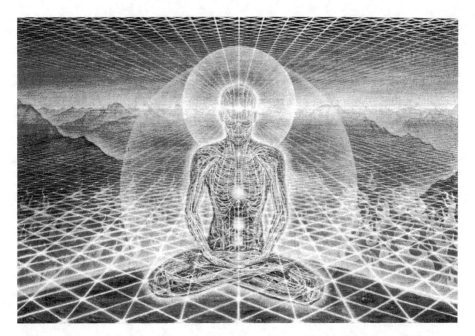

Alex Grey, *Theologue*. Look at this powerful image, and see the nodes of light and the intersecting lines. See them as surrounding the living earth, with you as one intersection.

one point in the web in perfect peace. As you glimpse yourself as a healing artist and hold your healing vision, you help make the web and She is born.

Look at the Alex Grey painting Theologue, *and see the nodes of light and the intersecting lines. See them as surrounding the living earth, with you as one intersection. Hold your image or poem or song or healing prayer and make it your point of light. See the web as whole and you are seen and She is born again. Let this image flow around the earth and see yourself as one node, with your art and prayers as your emanation. Put yourself in the web and hold your vision of yourself as a healing artist with your vision that you are working on in place. See all the others around you as far as they go back and forward in time and space. Feel yourself heal, feel us heal, feel the earth heal.*

Go deeper now. Drop into your center. If you have healing forces, ancient spirits, or power animals, call them to you. Know that you are a healing artist who has a vision to heal yourself, others, and the earth. Feel deeply that as you hold this vision or even hold your space with intent, your node is lit up and radiates love and you make the web that heals the earth at this moment. Come out slowly, move your body, touch the ground, pray or meditate on peace, and go on with your day.

SEEING MORE OF THE VISION

In our vision, the path of the healing artist goes like this: 1. Creative healing: we let our images come out to heal and be seen. 2. The path of the feather: we let the earth speak to us; her voice becomes sacred again and we hear the voice of the ancient spirits and of the spirit animals. 3. The medicine wheel web: The medicine wheel emerges and the healing rituals are formed. Art and healing become one on earth.

Creative healing is actually about the way people see the visions that come from within them and begin to use them with intent to heal. So it is the first step. It is the beginning of how you find out who you are, how you find out your story, how you heal yourself, how you heal others and the earth. It is only after you start to use your images to heal that your creativity becomes illuminated and you can move from the ordinary world into an extraordinary world, one that can be a more visionary world. In the visionary world, your images are formed in color, light, and movement; spirit animals come, and magical landscapes and ancient ancestral spirits appear. Spirit guides like She Who Gardens Us from Above become a part of your creative and visionary life. You can hear the music, the words, the art from the inner world that is at once magical, mystical, and mysterious. Then you as the artist healer become the contemporary shaman who can hear Her song to heal the earth. This is when the "path of the feather" appears, and we see that the sacred sites and spirit animals call out to be heard by everyone. The medicine wheel web forms and shows us that if we all join around the earth as the noospere and see the same vision, the earth will be healed. Then all of you become the ones who heal the earth.

When we interviewed the healing artists for this book, we asked them how they ended up where they are. We asked them how they thought they ended up as healing artists when they started as studio artists or nurses or physicians. We were given two types of answers to our question. The first response was, "It is destiny. I am part of an ancient family; we have always sung Her story to heal the earth." The second answer was, "It is who I am, deeply who I am. By becoming a healing artist I am becoming myself." In a real sense, the two answers are the same, for as we join the ancient tradition of artists to heal the earth, we find out who we are.

A FINAL INVOCATION FOR OUR HEALING WORK TO BE DONE

Like the prayer that started this book, this is a small prayer to the forces that help us do our creative healing. Just as we called them in at the beginning of the book, we thank them and release them at the end.

God, Great Spirit, She Who Gardens Us from Above, we thank you for art and healing and for our lives. We thank you for the lives of our families; we thank you for the lives of the people with illnesses and the healing artists whom we talked to for this book. We thank you for this sacred work and for letting us do it. And we pray to you, we dream deeply up into Her heart that art and healing become one on earth. We dream deeply up into Her heart that art and healing will heal ourselves, others, and the earth. We dream deeply up into Her heart that art and healing will give each of us a reason for being, will change our lives into manifesting the full brilliance of who we are, and will allow us to love each other.

Art is a way of healing, art is a way of knowing, art is a way of caring.

BIBLIOGRAPHY

Journal Articles about Art and Healing

Aldridge, D. 1994. An overview of music therapy research. *Complementary Therapies in Medicine.*

Amonite, D. W. 1996. The role of art therapy as an emotional support system for HIV/AIDS-related issues. *International Conference on AIDS* Jul 7–12; 11(2): 428 (abstract no. Th.D.5155).

Antonovsky, A. 1984. A sense of coherence as a determinant of health. *Behavioral Health.*

Bandura, A. 1985. Catecholamine secretion as a function of perceived coping; self-efficacy. *Journal of Consulting and Clinical Psychology* 53(3): 406.

Breslow, D. M. 1993. Creative arts for hospitals: the UCLA experiment. *Patient-Educ-Couns* Jun; 21(1–2): 101–10.

Bruck, L. 1994. Nursing care; artists-in-residence. *Nursing Homes* Sep; 43(7): 50–51.

Byers, J. F., and K. A. Smyth. 1997. Effect of a music intervention on noise annoyance, heart rate, and blood pressure in cardiac surgery patients. *American Journal on Critical Care* May; 6(3): 183–91.

Caudell, K. A. 1996. Psychoneuroimmunology and innovative behavioral interventions in patients with leukemia. *Oncology Nursing Forum* Apr; 23(3): 493–502.

Covington, H., and C. Crosby. 1997. Music therapy as a nursing intervention. *Journal Psychosoc-Nurs-Mental Health Services* Mar; 35(3): 34–37.

Dossey, L. 1988. The rediscovery of the mind. *Advances* 5(3): 73.

Dubois, J. M., T. Bartter, and M. R. Pratter. 1995. Music improves patient comfort level during outpatient bronchoscopy. *Chest: The Cardiopulmonary Journal* Jul; 108(1): 129–30.

Fawzy, I. Malignant melanoma: effects of an early stractired psychiatric intervention coping and affective state on recurrence and survival six years later. *Archives of General Psychiatry* 50(681): 9.

Good, M. 1996. Effects of relaxation and music on postoperative pain: a review. *Journal of Advanced Nursing* Nov; 24(5): 905–14.

Graham-Pole, J., M. R. Lane, M. L. Kitakis, and L. Stacpoole. 1996. Re-storying lives, restoring selves: the arts and healing, Gainesville June 22–25, 1995. Symposium IJAM. *International Journal of Arts Medicine (IJAM)* 4(1): 20–23.

Hall, H. R. 1983. Hypnosis and the immune system. *Journal of Clinical Hypnosis* 25(2): 92.

Henry, L. L. 1995. Music therapy: a nursing intervention for the control of pain and anxiety in the ICU: a review of the research literature. *Dimensions of Critical Care Nursing* Nov-Dec; 14(6): 295–304.

Hoffman, J. 1997. Alternatives: complementary therapies; tuning in to the power of music. *RN* Jun; 60(6): 52–54, 57.

Johnston, K., and J. Rohaly-Davis. 1996. An introduction to music therapy: helping the oncology patient in the ICU. *Critical Care Nurse Quarterly* Feb; 18(4): 54–60.

Kobasa, S. Personality and constitution as mediators in the stress-illness relationship. *Journal of Health and Social Behavior* 22: 368.

Lane, M. T., and J. Graham-Pole. 1994. Development of an art program on a bone marrow transplant unit. *Cancer Nurse* Jun; 17(3): 185–92.

———. 1994. The power of creativity in healing: a practice model demonstrating the links between the creative arts and the art of nursing. *NLN Publication* Jun; (14–26): 203–22.

Lelievre, D. 1996. Art therapy support groups conceived in an integrative way: a global approach for reinforcing self-esteem of people living with HIV/AIDS. *International Conference on AIDS* Jul 7–12; 11(1): 406 (abstract no. Tu.D.2851).

Lindsay, S. 1993. Dec 15–1994, Jan 18. Music in hospitals. *British Journal of Hospital Medicine;* 50(11): 660–62.

Lynn, D. 1995. Healing through art, art-therapy. *Journal of the American Art Therapy Association* 12(1): 70–71.

McIntyre, B. B. 1988. Art therapy in hospice care. *Caring* Aug; 7(8): 48–49.

McKinney, C. H., F. C. Tims, A. Kumar, and M. Kumar. 1997. The effect of selected classical music and spontaneous imagery on plasma beta-endorphin. *Journal on Behavioral Medicine* Feb; 20(1): 85–99.

Magill-Levreault, L. 1993. Music therapy in pain and symptom management. *Journal of Palliative Care* Winter; 9(4): 42–48.

Malchiodi, C. A. 1993. Medical art therapy: contributions to the field of arts medicine. *International Journal of Arts Medicine (IJAM)* Fall; 2(2): 28–31.

Oldham, J. 1989. Psychological support for cancer patients. *British Journal of Occupational Therapy* Dec; 52(12): 463–65.

Pelletier, K., and D. Herzing. 1988. Psychoneuroimmunology: toward a mind-body model. *Advances* 5(1): 27.

Perlis, C., D. Wallace, and E. Rosenbaum. 1994. Sharing the patient experience in the classroom with the Art For Recovery program. (AFR) (meeting abstract). *Proc-Annual Meeting of the American Society of Clinical Oncologists.* 13: A1552 Predeger-E.

Pert, C. 1986. The wisdom of the receptors: neuropeptides, the emotions, and bodymind. *Advances* 3(3): 8.

Roche, J. 1992. Spiritual care of the person with AIDS: Literature and art can touch closed hearts. *Health Prog* Mar; 73(2): 78–81.

Sabo, C. E., and S. R. Michael. 1996. The influence of personal message with music on anxiety and side effects associated with chemotherapy. *Cancer Nursing* Aug; 19(4): 283–89.

Sambandham, M., and V. Schirm. 1995. Music as a nursing intervention for residents with Alzheimer's disease in long-term care. *Geriatric Nursing* Mar-Apr; 16(2): 79–83.

Samuels, M. 1995. Art as a healing force. *Alternative Therapies in Health and Medicine* Sep; 1(4): 38–40.

———. 1993. Art as a healing force: an essay. *Bolinas Museum Catalog.*

Schneider, J., et al. 1983. The relationship of mental imagery to white blood cell (neutrophil) function. Uncirculated mimeograph, Michigan State University College of Medicine.

Schroeder-Sheker, T. 1994. Music for the dying: a personal account of the new field of music-thanatology—history, theories, and clinical narratives. *Journal of Holistic Nursing* Mar; 12(1): 83–99.

Sonke-Henderson, J. 1996. Healing through art. *Women's Health Digest* 2(4): 330–31.

Sourkes, B. M. 1991. Truth to life: art therapy with pediatric oncology patients and their siblings. *Journal Psychosoc. Oncology* 9(2): 81–96.

Spiegel, David, et al. 1989. Effect of psychosocial treatment on survival of women with metastatic breast cancer. *Lancet* 2(8668): 881–91.

Standley, J. M., and S. B. Hanser. 1995. Music therapy research and applications in pediatric oncology treatment. *Journal of Pediatric Oncology Nursing* Jan; 12(1): 3–8; discussion 9–10.

Stern, R. S. 1989. Many ways to grow: creative art therapies. *Pediatric Annals* 645: 649–52.

Sundaram, R. 1995. In focus: art therapy with a hospitalized child. *American Journal of Art Therapy: Art in Psychotherapy Rehabilitation and Education* Aug; 34(1): 2–8.

Updike, P. 1990. Music therapy results for ICU patients. *Dimensions of Critical Care Nursing* 9: 39–45.

———. 1990. Through the lens of the artist-scientist: reflections for the pediatric oncology nurse. *Journal of Pediatric Oncology Nursing* 7(1): 4–8.

Walker, C. 1989. Use of art and play therapy in pediatric oncology. *Journal of Pediatric Oncology Nursing* Oct; 6(4): 121–26.

Watkins, G. R. 1997. Music therapy: proposed physiological mechanisms and clinical implications. *Clinical Nurse Specialist* Mar; 11(2): 43–50.

Ziesler, A. A. 1993. Art therapy—a meaningful part of cancer care. *Journal of Cancer Care* Apr; 2(2): 107–11.

Zimmerman, L., J. Nieveen, S. Barnason, and M. Schmaderer. 1996. The effects of music interventions on postoperative pain and sleep in coronary artery bypass graft (CABG) patients . . . including commentary by Miaskowski. C *Scholarly Inquiry for Nursing Practice* Summer; 10(2): 153–74.

Books about Art and Healing

Achterberg, J. *Using Imagery for Health and Wellness.* 1994.

———. *Imagery and Healing.* Shambhala, 1985.

Ader, R. *Psychoneuroimmunology.* Academia Press, 1981.

Allan, P. B. *Art Is a Way of Knowing: A Guide to Self-Knowledge and Spiritual Fulfillment through Creating.* Shambhala, 1995.

Arieh, S. *Creativity: The Magic Synthesis.* Basic Books, 1976.

Audette, A. H. *The Blank Canvas: Inviting the Muse.* Shambhala, 1993.

Blofeld, J. *The Tantric Mysticism of Tibet.* Prajna Press, 1970.

Bolle, K. *The Bhagavadgita.* Univ. of California Press, 1979.

Borysenko, J. *Minding the Body, Mending the Mind.* Addison-Wesley, 1987.

Cameron, J. *The Vein of Gold: A Journey to Your Creative Heart.* Jeremy P. Tarcher/Putnam, 1996.

Campbell, D. *The Mozart Effect.* 1996.

———. *The Roar of Silence.* Theosophical Publishing House, 1989.

Campbell, J. *The Hero with a Thousand Faces.*

———. *The Inner Reaches of Outer Space.* Alfred Van Der Marck, 1986.

———. *The Masks of God: Oriental Mythology.* Penguin, 1976.

———. *The Masks of God: Primitive Mythology.* Penguin, 1976.

———. *Myths to Live By.* Bantam Books, 1973.

Campbell, J., R. Eisler, M. Gimbutas, and C. Muses. *In All Her Names.* Harper Collins Publishers, 1993.

Cassou, M., and Stewart Cubley. *Life, Paint and Passion: Reclaiming the Magic of Spontaneous Expression.* Putnam, 1993.

Castaneda, C. *The Eagle's Gift.* Pocket Books, 1981.

Chodorow, J. *Dance Therapy and Depth Psychology: The Moving Imagination.* Routledge, 1991.

Cornell, J. *Drawing the Light from Within: Keys to Awaken Your Creative Power.* Quest Books, 1997.

Edwards, B. *Drawing on the Artist Within.* Simon & Schuster, Inc., 1986.

———. *Drawing on the Right Side of the Brain.* J. P. Tarcher, 1989.

Eliade, M. *Myths, Dreams, and Mysteries.* Harper & Row, 1957.

———. *Rites and Symbols of Initiation.* Harper & Row, 1958.

———. *The Sacred and the Profane.* Harcourt Brace & World, 1957.

———. *Shamanism.* Princeton Univ. Press, 1972.

———. *The Two and the One.* Harper & Row, 1969.

———. *Yoga Immortality and Freedom.* Pantheon, 1958.

Evans-Evans Wentz, W. Y. *Tibetan Yoga and Secret Doctrines.* Oxford Univ. Press, 1958.

Fox, M. *The Coming of the Cosmic Christ.* Harper & Row, 1988.

Gablik. S. *The Reenchantment of Art.* New York: Thames and Hudson, 1991.

Gardner, Kay. *Sounding the Inner Landscape*. Caduceus Publications, 1990.

Ghiselin, B. *The Creative Process: A Symposium*. Univ. of California Press, 1953.

Goldberg, N. *Living Color: A Writer Paints Her World*. Bantam Books, 1997.

———. *Writing Down to the Bones*. Shambala, 1986.

Grey, A. *Sacred Mirrors*. Inner Traditions International, 1990.

Guzzetta, C. E. Music therapy: hearing the melody of the soul. In B. M. Dossey, et al. (eds.), *Holistic Nursing: A Handbook for Practice* 2d ed. Aspen Publishing, 1995.

Halprin, A. *Moving toward Life*. Wesleyan University Press, 1995.

———. *Dance as a Healing Art*. Tamalpa Institute, 1997.

Harner, M. *The Way of the Shaman*. Bantam Books, 1982.

Harvey, A. *The Way of Passion: A Celebration of Rumi*. Frog Ltd., 1994.

Highwater, J. *Dance Rituals of Experience*. A. W. Publishers, 1978.

Jacobson, E. *How to Relax and Have Your Baby*. McGraw-Hill, 1965.

Jahn, G. *Margins of Reality*. Harcourt Brace Jovanovich, 1987.

Jung, C. *Man and His Symbols*. Doubleday & Co., 1964.

———. *Memories, Dreams, Reflections*. Vintage Books, 1961.

Justice, B. *Who Gets Sick*. Tarcher, 1987.

Kandinsky, W. *Concerning the Spiritual in Art*. Translated and with an introduction by M. T. H. Sadler. Dover, 1977.

Klaus, M., and J. Kennell. *Parent-Infant Bonding*. C. V. Mosby, 1982.

Krup, M. *Current Medical Diagnosis and Treatment*. Appleton and Lang, 1997.

Lane, M. T. Model of creativity. In P. Chinn (ed.), *Art and Aesthetics in Nursing*. National League for Nursing, 1994.

Lee, R., and I. DeVore. *Kalahari Hunter-Gatherers*. Harvard Univ. Press, 1976.

LeShan, L. *Cancer as a Turning Point*. E. P. Dutton, 1989.

Levine, S. *Meetings at the Edge*. Doubleday and Co., 1974.

Locke, S. *The Healer Within*. New American Library, 1986.

Lovelock, J. E. *Gaia*. Oxford Univ. Press, 1979.

Luthe, W. *Autogenic Therapy*. Grune & Stratton, 1970.

McNiff, S. *Art as Medicine*. Shambhala, 1992.

Maisel, E. *Affirmations for Artists*. Jeremy P. Tarcher/Putnam, 1996.

Metzger, D. *Writing for Your Life: A Guide and Companion to the Inner Worlds*. Harper Collins, 1992.

Muktananda, S. *Meditate*. State Univ. of New York Press, 1980.

Ornstein, R., and D. Sobel. *The Healing Brain*. Simon and Schuster, 1987.

Oyle, I. *The Healing Mind*. Celestial Arts, 1974.

Rogers, N. *The Creative Connection*. Science and Behavior Books, 1993.

Rossman, M. *Healing Yourself*. Walker and Co., 1987.

Samuels, M., and H. Bennett. *Be Well*. Random House-Bookworks, 1974.

———. *Spirit Guides*. Random House-Bookworks, 1973.

———. *The Well Body Book*. Random House-Bookworks, 1972.

———. *Well Body, Well Earth*. Sierra Club, 1982.

Samuels, M., and N. Samuels. *Healing with the Mind's Eye*. Summit Books, 1990.

———. *Seeing with the Mind's Eye*. Random House-Bookworks, 1975.

———. *The Well Adult*. Summit Books, 1988.

Siegel, B. *Love, Medicine and Miracles*. Harper & Row, 1986.

Simonton, S., and C. Simonton. *Getting Well Again*. Bantam Books, 1978.

Swimme, B. *The Universe Is a Green Dragon*. Bear & Co., 1984.

Tart, C. *Altered States of Consciousness*. Doubleday and Co., 1972.

Van Manen, M. *Researching the Lived Experience*. Human Science for an Action Sensitive Pedagogy, 1990.

Wilhelm, R. *The Secret of the Golden Flower*. Routledge & Kegan Paul, 1969.

Woodman, M. *Addiction to Perfection*. Inner City Books, 1982.

Wyngaarden, J. *Cecil Textbook of Medicine*. W. B. Saunders, 1996.

ABOUT THE AUTHORS

The coauthors of *Creative Healing* both have extensive personal and professional experiences with art and healing.

Michael Samuels, M.D., has used art and guided imagery with cancer patients for over twenty-five years in private practice and in consultation. He has watched as his patients have drawn, played music, and written themselves well. He is on the advisory boards of Commonweal (for their cancer retreats) and Tamalpa Institute, an organization that uses dance for healing. He also experienced the power of art and healing personally as he wrote a journal and a novel while his wife lived and then died with breast cancer. He found that his writing was the major healing intervention he did during that difficult period. It kept him positive and helped him love her in the most stressful time. He is also the cofounder and director of Art As A Healing Force, a project started in 1990 and devoted to making art and healing one. He lectures and does nationwide workshops for physicians, nurses, artists, and patients on how to use art in healing. He has organized many nationwide conferences on art and healing and visits and participates in projects in hospitals where art and music are used with patients. He networks people in the field and is a recognized leader in art and healing. He is the author of fourteen books, including the best-selling *Well Body Book, Well Baby Book, Well Pregnancy Book,* and *Seeing with the Mind's Eye.* He lives in Bolinas, California, and has two grown sons.

Mary Rockwood Lane, R.N., M.S.N., Ph.D. cand., is a painter and a nurse. She experienced art and healing firsthand as she painted herself out of a severe depression. With what she learned in that experience, she became the cofounder and codirector of the Arts In Medicine program at the University of Florida, Gainesville, and founded their artist-in-residence program. She has led and developed that program for over five years, and she now is doing research in art and healing for her Ph.D. in nursing at the University of Florida, Gainesville.

Her Ph.D. thesis is on the patient's lived experience of art and healing, and the research for it is in progress. It will be the first advanced degree in art and healing in the nursing field. She has written many articles on art and healing in nursing and medical journals and is a recognized leader in the field. She lectures and teaches workshops on art and healing around the world and helps medical centers and artists set up art and healing programs. She lives in Gainesville, Florida, is married, and has three children.